Lecture Notes in Medical Informatics

Vol. 1: Medical Informatics Europe 78. Proceedings 1978. Edited by J. Anderson. XI, 822 pages. 1978.

Vol. 2: D. Fenna, S. Abrahamsson, S. O. Lööw and H. Peterson, The Stockholm County Medical Information System. VI, 163 pages. 1978.

Vol. 3: Long-Term Studies on Side-Effects of Contraception – State and Planning. Symposium 1977. Edited by U. Kellhammer and K. Überla. VI, 240 pages. 1978.

Vol. 4: Clinical Trials in 'Early' Breast Cancer. Proceedings 1978. Edited by H. R. Scheurlen, G. Weckesser and I. Armbruster. VI, 283 pages. 1979.

Vol. 5: Medical Informatics Berlin 1979. Proceedings 1979. Edited by B. Barber, F. Grémy, K. Überla and G. Wagner. XXIII, 970 pages. 1979.

Vol. 6: Health Care Technology Evaluation. Proceedings, 1978. Edited by J. Goldman. VII, 118 pages. 1979.

Vol. 7: Technology and Health: Man and his World. Proceedings, 1978. Edited by G. Wagner, P. L. Reichertz and E. Masè. VI, 243 pages. 1980.

Vol. 8: Mathematical Aspects of Computerized Tomography. Proceedings 1980. Edited by F. Natterer. VIII, 309 pages. 1981.

Vol. 9: Computers and Mathematical Models in Medicine. Proceedings, 1977. Edited by D. Cardús and C. Vallbona. VIII, 315 pages. 1981.

Vol. 10: B. Fries, Applications of Operations Research to Health Care Delivery Systems. V, 107 pages. 1981.

Vol. 11: Medical Informatics Europe 81. Proceedings 1981. Edited by F. Grémy, P. Degoulet, B. Barber, and R. Salamon. XXIII, 975 pages. 1981.

Vol. 12: G. Wiederhold, Databases for Health Care. VI, 75 pages. 1981.

Vol. 13: The Computer and Blood Banking. Proceedings, 1981. Edited by J. R. Möhr and A. Kluge. X, 275 pages. 1981.

Vol. 14.: F. Wingert, Medical Informatics. X, 247 pages. 1981.

Vol. 15: Digital Image Processing in Medicine. Proceedings 1981. Edited by K. H. Höhne. VIII, 197 pages. 1981.

Vol. 16: Medical Informatics Europe 82. Proceedings, 1982. Edited by R.R. O'Moore, B. Barber, P.L. Reichertz, and F. Roger. XX, 938 pages. 1982.

Vol. 17: Biomedical Images and Computers. Proceedings, 1980. Edited by J. Sklansky and J.-C. Bisconte. VII, 332 pages. 1982.

Vol. 18: D.P. Pretschner, Engymetry and Personal Computing in Nuclear Medicine. V, 129 pages. 1982.

Vol. 19: R.L. Blum, Discovery and Representation of Causal Relationships from a Large Time-Oriented Clinical Database: The RX Project. XIX, 242 pages. 1982.

Vol. 20: S. Biefang, W. Köpcke, M.A. Schreiber, Manual for the Planning and Implementation of Therapeutic Studies. V, 100 pages. 1983.

Vol. 21: Influence of Economic Instability on Health. Proceedings, 1981. Edited by J. John, D. Schwefel, and H. Zöllner. VIII, 528 pages. 1983.

Vol. 22: Objective Medical Decision-making; Systems Approach in Acute Disease. Proceedings, 1983. Edited by J. E W. Beneken and S.M. Lavelle. VIII, 243 pages. 1983.

Lecture Notes in Medical Informatics

Edited by P. L. Reichertz and D. A. B. Lindberg

29

System Analysis of Ambulatory Care in Selected Countries

– With Special Concern for Computer Support –

Edited by
P. L. Reichertz, R. Engelbrecht and U. Piccolo

Springer-Verlag
Berlin Heidelberg New York London Paris Tokyo

Editors

Peter L. Reichertz
Institut für Med. Informatik, Med. Hochschule Hannover
Konstanty-Gutschow-Straße 8, 3000 Hannover 61

Rolf Engelbrecht
MEDIS-Institut, Gesellschaft für Strahlen- und Umweltforschung mbH München
Ingolstädter Landstraße 1, 8042 Neuherberg

Ursula Piccolo
Institut für Med. Informatik, Med. Hochschule Hannover
Konstanty-Gutschow-Straße 8, 3000 Hannover 61

ISBN-13:978-3-540-17159-1 e-ISBN-13:978-3-642-93341-7
DOI: 10.1007/978-3-642-93341-7

2127/3140-543210

FOREWORD

The Working Group 5 of the International Medical Informatics Association (IMIA) is dedicated to information systems in primary care with special emphasis on computer systems in the doctor's office. Accordingly, a conference was held in Hannover in 1980 where the first approaches were described and experiences in system analysis, system construction and evaluation were discussed (Rienhoff, O. and Abrams, M.E. (eds.): The Computer in the Doctor's Office, North-Holland, Amsterdam: 1980).

Computer hardware and software development has been rapid over the last years. Thus the prerequisites for a successful support of the work of the physician in his office have improved. But system construction still lags behind and the actual penetration of systems is lower than 2 % of the doctors' offices in most countries. This applies to industrialized countries. However, attempts are made everywhere to improve primary care by means of modern information technology.

Information systems depend upon the real environment into which they are placed: administrative procedures govern priorities and procedures in doctor's office computers, possibilities to defray cost upon the various carriers or the patients have a great influence on the propagation of systems. Furthermore, various procedures of accounting or re-imbursement may lead to a facilitation or to a delay of the introduction of systems. The 'art of medical practice' has reached a comparable standard within at least the industrialized countries. Nonetheless, specific aspects of health care delivery vary. Therefore it is not possible to export one type of system to another country: many adjustments have to be made in order to meet the local requirements. Administrative and claim-processing procedures, most important e.g. in the Federal Republic of Germany, Switzerland, Austria, etc. are of no interest in countries with a national health system (like e.g. the United Kingdom). Therefore, the spectrum of system components varies. 'Medical components', e.g. those which directly support patient care, often have to be financed by administrative components, thus justifying the acquisition of a system. Furthermore, the way of delivering health care in primary care is of importance: single physicians' practices have less financial means than large group practices.

However, in many conferences systems are compared without considering these basic facts. Industry also tries to market systems, which have been successful in one country, in other countries and are disappointed when this attempt remains unsuccessful.

Therefore, the follow-up conference of the IMIA Working Group 5, held in Munich, December 2-6, 1985, dedicated one stream of discussions to the presentation of the system analysis of health care systems in selected countries: mostly those countries where activities can be seen in the field of introduction of information technology into ambulatory care. These presentations were meant to serve as the basis for the comparison of actual systems and concepts of technology development. During the conference, however, it became clear that the resulting collection of system analyses may also serve as a reference for other purposes: Discussions of the organization of health care in the various countries, schemes of re-imbursement, structural problems and general developments. It was therefore decided that the system analytical part of the conference should be published separately in order to be made available also to health administrators, planners,researchers and other people interested in general aspects of health care delivery.

The results of the more specific contributions to the conference (descriptions of actual systems, aspects of long-term documentation and patient care, expert systems in ambulatory care, new technologies and standardization, etc.) are published in a second volume in the same series.

Hopefully, this volume may serve as a general reference for information and will stimulate discussions on the varying structures of health care delivery in primary and ambulatory care.

The conference, held as an IMIA Working Conference, was co-sponsored by the World Health Organization (European Office), the Deutsche Forschungsgemeinschaft (DFG), the Gesellschaft für Strahlen- und Umweltforschung (GSF/München), the Medical School Hannover and supported by grants from the Deutscher Akademischer Austauschdienst (DAAD) and various federal and Bavarian ministries. To all these institutions we owe our thanks. Without their active and idealistic support we could not have achieved a conference which was characterized by vivid discussions and the exchange of many ideas. The organization was supported by Mrs. A. Heimers/Hannover and the local staff of the GSF in Munich.

Peter L. Reichertz
Rolf Engelbrecht
Ursula Piccolo

TABLE OF CONTENTS

TABLE OF CONTENTS

INFORMATION FOR PRIMARY HEALTH CARE - WHO'S VIEWPOINT

World Health Organization, H. Vuori, T. McKeown, The Swedish Ministry for Health and Social Affairs, Nordisk Medicinal-Statistisk Kommitté

Hannu Vuori, M.D., Ph.D., M.A., Chief, Research Promotion and Development, World Health Organization Regional Office for Europe, Scherfigsvej 8, 2100 Copenhagen

To be able to identify the information needs for and of primary health care, one needs to know what the concept means.

The current interest in primary health care (PHC) no doubt results from the push given to it by the World Health Organization (WHO). WHO views PHC as the key to achieving its overriding health policy goal "health for all by the year 2000" (HFA) (WHO 1977: Resolution WHA30.43). At the International Conference on Primary Health Care, the leading health authorities of some 140 countries approved the Alma-Ata Declaration, which lays down the principles of PHC (WHO/UNICEF 1978).

This paper describes the main facets of PHC as understood by WHO and identifies their information implications. It aims at answering the following questions: what does WHO mean with PHC; how does WHO want to develop PHC; and what do we need to know about PHC as seen by WHO. The WHO viewpoint results in certain biases related to the level of health care, user of information, type of data, and technology used:

- level: the focus is on the <u>system</u> as opposed to individual practices;
- user: the focus is on the needs of <u>administrators</u> and <u>planners</u> rather than those of individual providers of care;
- type of data: the focus is often more on <u>qualitative</u> than quantitative data; and
- technology: any device or method to collect and analyze data will do; there is no emphasis on computers or other technology.

WHAT IS PRIMARY HEALTH CARE?

Fallacies and problems

Fallacies: Given the solemn commitment given to PHC in Alma-Ata as well as the lip service paid to it and the wealth of material written about it, one would assume the concept to be unequivocal and clear. This is not the case. Particularly in the industrialized countries, one stumbles on three common fallacies (Vuori 1982, 1984a):

- primary health care is something new, invented at the Alma-Ata Conference and since propagated by WHO;

- primary health care is something for the developing countries ("poor care for poor people" as a distinguished hospital administrator put it), irrelevant for the needs of the industrialized countries; and

- primary <u>health</u> care is identical with primary <u>medical</u> care.

The fallacies are understandable but not justified. It is true that the term primary health care did not become a household word until after the Alma-Ata

Conference. The term had, however, been used by WHO and even by some member states long before and many of the principles of the Alma-Ata Declaration were embodied in such earlier WHO concepts as basic health services and comprehensive health services. The Alma-Ata Conference posited primary health care as an alternative to the current high technology and hospital oriented main stream of health care in the industrialized countries. It thus easily gave rise to the idea that primary health care is something new.

It is also true that the language of the Alma-Ata Declaration was chosen with the developing countries primarily in mind. It can therefore be easily misinterpreted as a new orientation, intended for developing countries.

The claim that primary medical care is identical with primary health care is particularly dear to those health authorities and health professionals who want to give the impression of being all for primary health care but who in fact are either opposed to it or have not quite understood what it means. It is easy to refer to the activities of the primary care physicians (usually but not always general practitioners), equate them with primary health care and then proceed to say that no further development of primary health care is needed.

Problems: Even if one manages to prove that the three fallacies are just fallacies, the development of primary health care in Europe is still fraught with problems. They can be grouped under the following headings: conceptual; political and attitudinal; organizational; managerial; and training problems.

Conceptual problems primarily result from lacking comprehension of the overall ramifications of the Alma-Ata approach to primary health care; more often than not, the concept is understood too narrowly. The result is the false equation of primary medical care with primary health care. The definition of primary medical care varies from country to country. Sometimes it is defined on the basis of types of health problems (trivial versus complicated), sometimes types of providers (general practitioners versus specialists) and sometimes again on the basis of types of health care facility providing services (health centres or polyclinics versus hospitals).

All told, the health politicians, health authorities, health professionals and the public have difficulties in taking seriously a concept which seems to be vaguely defined and whose contents seem to change from country to country and situation to situation.

The political problems are related to the fact that at least till today, primary health care has been deemed politically less prestigious than specialized, hospital based care. The resources given to primary health care are a tiny fraction of those devoted to secondary and tertiary care; in many countries as little as 5 to 10 per cent of total health care budget goes to primary care. Consequently - as the essence of politics is the control of resources and the power derived from this control - very few politicians venture to make the promotion of primary care the basis of their health policy platform.

Attitudinal problems can be found particularly among the health professionals. The educational tradition, particularly that of physicians, is geared to hospital based medicine. It equates high quality with disease orientation, curative work, hospitals and specialization. Health professionals derive more emotional and intellectual satisfaction from specialized care than from primary care, which seldom offers such thrills as, for instance, major surgery. One also has to admit that the scientific basis of prevention and health promotion is not as solid as that of treatment or, in particular, that of diagnostic work. It is therefore understandable that the medical world still looks with, at worst, suspicion and, at best, curiosity at primary care.

Also the consumers' attitudes are often suspicious. It has demanded and got sophisticated high-technology medicine and has looked askance at primary care, often equating "primary" with "primitive". In all fairness to the public, one should add that it has not invented this attitude; it has just adopted the prevailing professional prejudices.

Organizational problems derive from the fact that in many European countries, there is no official system for primary health care, primary medical services being provided for by private practitioners in an uncoordinated fashion. This "non-system" may result in a biased geographical and socioeconomic distribution of the services and in an emphasis on curative services. Social and health services are often poorly integrated. Social services are often provided for by volontary or state agencies without any coordination or collaboration with the predominantly private primary medical care sector. Also the boundaries between lay care and professional health services are unclear.

The managerial problems are a corollary of the previous ones. As the primary health care system as a whole is, in many countries, poorly defined, it has not been possible or it has not been felt necessary to develop effective managerial structures and techniques, nor to include managerial aspects in the training of health professionals.

The training problems are easy to summarize: the current training of health professionals is inadequate for primary health care. It imparts wrong knowledge, skills and attitudes; it is given in the wrong place by wrong people.

Four facets of PHC

The Alma-Ata Declaration defines PHC as follows (WHO 1978):

> Primary health care is essential health care made universally accessible to individuals and families in the community by means acceptable to them, through their full participation and at a cost that the community and country can afford. It forms an integral part both of the country's health system of which it is the nucleus and of the overall social and economic development of the community.

This is more a description of certain desirable characteristics of a system than an unequivocal definition of an important concept. It can be made more concrete and operational by distinguishing four facets or interpretations of PHC (Vuori 1984a and b):

- primary health care as a set of activities;
- primary health care as a level of care;
- primary health care as a strategy of organizing health care; and
- primary health care as a philosophy.

Primary health care as a set of activities: This is the most down-to-earth interpretation. The Alma-Ata Declaration states that primary health care involves at least:

- health education;
- food supply and proper nutrition;
- safe water and basic sanitation;
- maternal and child health care;
- immunization;
- prevention and control of endemic diseases;
- basic treatment of health problems; and
- provision of essential drugs.

According to this interpretation, one could say that a country has primary health care if its health care system includes these eight basic elements. This interpretation is simple and concrete but it also easily gives rise to the claims concerning the irrelevance of primary health care for the industrialized countries. One often hears health authorities and professionals say: "We already have all this; we have in fact had it since the beginning of the century." This claim is incorrect. One only needs to look, for example, at the immunization status of the population or social class and regional differences in infant mortality within a country, to realize that we still have problems that are amenable to solution by better primary health care. The minimum services can also be organized without any attention to the principles contained in the three other interpretations of primary health care.

Primary health care as a level of care: This too is an easily comprehensible interpretation of PHC. It is that part of the care system which the population contacts first when it has health problems. In many countries the situation seems to be quite clear: the first contact level comprises general practitioners, possibly public health nurses, home health visitors and other similar categories of health personnel. The problems begin, however, when one looks at the options. Perhaps up to 80-90% of all health related problems are being taken care of outside of the official health care system by the lay health care system. Is this part of the primary health care system? Are first contact visits to specialists or hospital out-patient departments also part of primary health care? And again, the first contact services can be organized completely disregarding the strategic or philosophical implications of the two remaining interpretations.

Primary health care as a strategy: This interpretation means that before one can speak of primary health care in a given country, the health services have to be organized taking certain strategic principles into account. The services have to be:

- accessible;
- relevant to the needs of the population;
- functionally integrated;
- based on community participation;
- cost-effective; and
- characterized by intersectorial collaboration.

In addition, a new distribution of resources between primary, secondary and tertiary health care may be needed as well as reorientation of health personnel both in their numbers, training and activities towards primary health care. This reorientation, in turn, may require legislative reforms enabling or facilitating a new division of labour and delegation of tasks. Many of these changes are a challenge to the current planning and management mechanisms. Consequently, they have to be strengthened and reoriented towards PHC.

Primary health care as a philosophy: This interpretation is the real raison d'être for WHO to be interested in primary health care. A country can claim to have primary health care in the most profound sense of the word only if its health care system is characterized by:

- social justice and equality;
- self-responsibility;
- international solidarity; and
- acceptance of a broad concept of health.

In the developing countries it has become painfully clear that it is impossible to guarantee the right to health - a principle included in the constitution of many newly independent countries - of every citizen by means of sophisticated high-technology medicine. Even the industrialized countries have reached an impasse: no country is rich enough to offer all of its citizens with everything that modern medicine can offer. In addition, at times of slow economic growth a hard look has to be taken at the cost-effectiveness of health care. The marginal utility of many of the latest innovations has been found to be low. The consequence has been an attempt to find alternatives that would be socially acceptable, cost-effective and affordable. The suggested solution is primary health care. It is the only way to bring about social equity in front of disease.

The concept of international solidarity simply means the extension of the principle of social justice beyond national boundaries to cover international collaboration. The rich countries owe it to the poor ones to help them to develop a health care system based on PHC. One effective form of help is to demonstrate clearly that the industrialized countries too believe in primary health care and take it seriously.

The concept of self-responsibility is one of the cornerstones of primary health care. With the increasing recognition of the role of human behaviour in the pathogenesis, it has been realized that an individual can - and should - do much more for his own health. Mothers, other family members, friends and other lay people can contribute a lot. The society should naturally help the individual in his attempts. Rather than making his task that of a modern Sisyphos who has to fight against obstacles such as adverse price policy and advocation of lifestyles conducive to poor health, the society should - to use a WHO slogan - "make the healthy choice the easy choice".

Studies (e.g. McKeown 1976), experience and common sense suggest that the official health care and health services are a minor determinant only of the actual health status of the population. A broad concept of health and its determinants is needed. A prime example is the current scourge of many industrialized societies: unemployment. The health care system can do very little about this and many other health hazards. Consequently, collaboration with other sectors of the society is needed.

Four facets rather than four interpretations: To summarize, none of the four interpretations suffices alone; primary health care is a broad concept having four facets rather than a concept that can be interpreted in four different ways. All the facets have to be present before one can speak of true primary health care: PHC is a set of activities, a level of care, a strategy to organizing health services and a philosophy permeating the entire health care system. Consequently no one group of health professionals or lay people can monopolize it; it is a team effort.

HOW TO DEVELOP PRIMARY HEALTH CARE?

Where do we stand?

When developing primary health care one has to start from the existing situation. When asked, most national health authorities or representatives of the health professionals in Europe would probably define primary health care in their country as the primary medical care system, consisting of general practitioners, front line specialists (usually general internists, general surgeons, pediatricians, gynaecologists and oto-rhino-laryngologists) and possibly some other categories of health personnel working either singlehandedly in private practices, or as teams in health centres, polyclinics or out-patient departments. There are four basic approaches with countless variations to organizing these services (fig. 1; Vuori 1980).

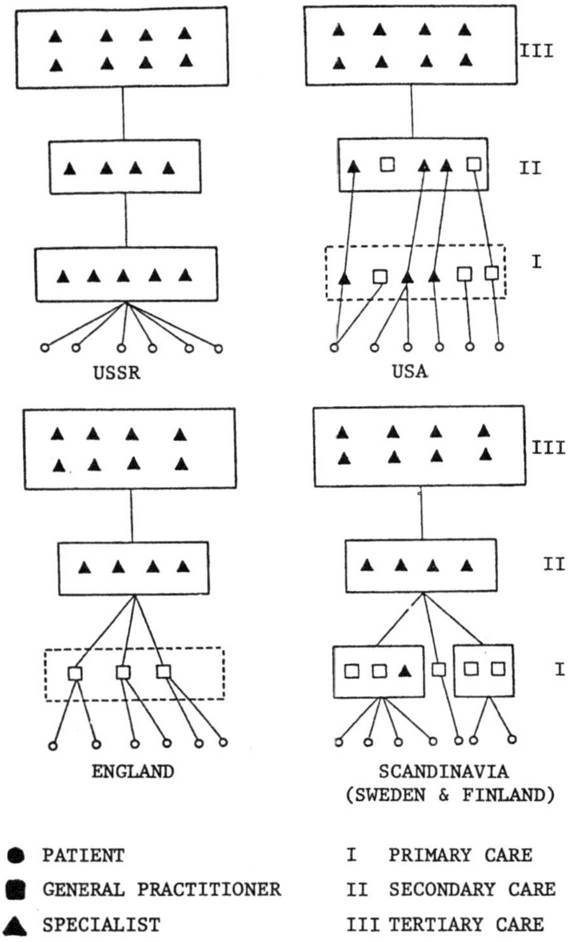

Fig. 1. Four basic models of primary medical care

In the socialist countries, virtually the entire population is covered by polyclinics, which in densely populated areas can be very large, providing facilities for up to fifty physicians, the majority of whom are specialists. In sparsely populated areas, the polyclinics are smaller and one also encounters general practitioners working alone. In the most remote areas auxiliaries may provide the first-contact services.

Many central European countries have a variant of the United States' model which consists of a relatively uncoordinated system of general practitioners working independently, either singly or in group practice. Other personnel categories may exist but they can rather be considered doctors' helpers than independent providers of health care.

In the British approach (National Health Service), a general practitioner is typically responsible for a group of patients who have chosen him as their primary care physician. In the Scandinavian system (Finland and Sweden), the focal point for the provision of care is not the general practitioner but a health centre run by the local administrative unit. The area of responsibility is not defined by the people's choice but by administrative boundaries. The personnel working in the health centres are salaried employees.

Another way to classify the current systems is to look at, on the one hand, whether they are public or private and, on the other hand, whether they are hospital or locally based (Fig. 2; Swedish Ministry of Health and Social Affairs 1981).

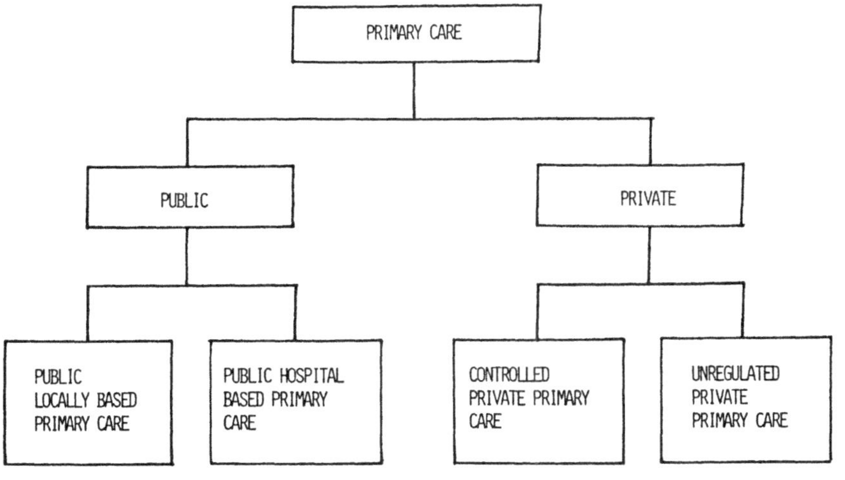

Fig. 2. Options for organizing primary care

It is probably safe to say that only public, locally based systems can cover all the four facets of primary health care; all other options are likely to be wanting in some respect and could more appropriately be called primary medical care.

Where to go?

Most of the systems in the European Member States of WHO are systems of primary medical care. Consequently, the main objective of WHO is to initiate and encourage in the Member States development which expands these systems towards primary health care. This development entails changes related to focus, contents, organization of, and responsibility for, health care (Table 1; Vuori 1984a and b).

If one is willing to take a critical look at the health care system of his country, one will easily realize what actions this blueprint suggests. The relative importance of the necessary changes depends on the situation in a given country. The blueprint has major implications for the information needed for PHC.

Table 1. From primary medical to primary health care

	From	To
Focus	ILLNESS CURE	HEALTH PREVENTION AND CARE
Contents	TREATMENT EPISODIC CARE SPECIFIC PROBLEMS	HEALTH PROMOTION CONTINUOUS CARE COMPREHENSIVE CARE
Organization	SPECIALISTS PHYSICIANS SINGLEHANDED PRACTICE	GENERAL PRACTITIONERS OTHER PERSONNEL GROUPS TEAM
Responsibility	HEALTH SECTOR ALONE PROFESSIONAL DOMINANCE PASSIVE RECEPTION	INTERSECTORIAL COLLABORATION COMMUNITY PARTICIPATION SELF-RESPONSIBILITY

WHAT DO WE NEED TO KNOW?

The question "what do we need to know?" can be divided into two subquestions (Vuori 1984c):

- information about primary health care: what do the international organizations and central, regional and local level health authorities of the Member States know about the current status and development of PHC; what do they need to know to be able to plan and develop it further?
- information for primary health care: what should those within the primary health care system, the providers of care, know about their own work; what additional information do they need to be able to perform their activities; and how do they get this information.

Given the WHO bias mentioned earlier, the focus will be on the information about PHC. Much of this information will also be relevant for the providers of care.

A social obligation to evaluate

Primary health care is a social experiment. It has been advocated as a solution to the alleged crisis of health care. Its promotion is, however, often based more on faith than on solid evidence. Is it indeed more cost-effective and socially acceptable than secondary and tertiary care; is it indeed more relevant to the needs of the population? These claims may be true but they cannot be accepted at face value. They have to be verified to establish the credibility of PHC in the eyes of health politicians, health professionals and the population at large. Similarly, the adversaries of PHC have put forward arguments that have not been tested or in whose support only anecdotal evidence exists; "lowering the quality of health care" and "turning the clock backwards" are typical examples. They also have to be tested (Vuori 1985).

Thus, if primary health care is the "key to attaining health for all" and the cornerstone of the health policies of the Member States it has to be evaluated. Two questions have to be answered: has primary health care been implemented and has it achieved its objectives.

WHO and monitoring of HFA

WHO takes the evaluation obligation seriously. The Alma-Ata Declaration (WHO 1978) emphasizes that in order to plan and manage primary health care the right kind of information is essential, but the collection of information has to be kept to the minimum required. PHC is, however, not a goal per se but an instrument to achieve HFA. Consequently, monitoring PHC is a part of the overall process of monitoring HFA.

The monitoring of HFA has developed stepwise. The first step in translating the overall goal of health for all into more operational terms was the global strategy (WHO 1981a). According to this Strategy, to permit governments to know whether they are making progress toward attaining an acceptable level of health for all their people, it is important that they introduce at the earliest stages a process of evaluation. This will include the assessment of the effectiveness and impact of the measures they are taking, and the monitoring of the progress and efficiency with which these measures are being carried out.

The next step consisted of adopting a set of 12 global indicators (WHO 1981a and b). One of them is directly related to PHC: the number of countries in which primary health care is available to the whole population, with at least the following:

- safe water in the home or within 15 minutes' walking distance, and adequate sanitary facilities in the home or immediate vicinity;
- immunization against diphtheria, tetanus, whooping cough, measles, poliomyelitis, and tuberculosis;
- local health care, including availability of at least 20 essential drugs, within one hour's walk or travel; and
- trained personnel for attending pregnancy and childbirth, and caring for children up to at least 1 year of age.

For the industrialized European Region, the global targets are too general. In addition, virtually all Member States have already achieved them. Consequently, the Regional Office first developed a Regional Strategy, adopted by the Regional Committee in 1980 (WHO 1980) and then Regional Targets in Support of HFA, adopted in 1984 (WHO 1984a).

The regional strategy states that to support planning, management and evaluation activities, countries will need more comprehensive and more specific health and health-related information. There will also have to be an agreed set of indicators. One of the targets specifically requests that before 1990, Member States should have health information systems capable of supporting their national strategies for health for all. Such systems should provide support for the planning, monitoring and evaluation of health development and services, assessment of national, regional and global progress towards health for all and dissemination of relevant scientific information.

The Member States have not shied away from their social obligation to monitor their efforts to achieve HFA. In connection with the regional targets, the European Regional Committee endorsed a set of 65 "essential" indicators and 43 "optional" indicators and "urged the Member States when reporting to the Regional Director, as far as possible to provide all the necessary information on progress and effectiveness in implementing their strategies for health for all, and in particular data related to the global and essential regional indicators" (WHO 1984b; resolution EUR/RC34/R5). In 1985, the first evaluation based on these indicators was presented to the Regional Committee (WHO 1985).

Information needed

After the above broad picture about monitoring the achievement of HFA, one can turn back to the specific information needs related to evaluating primary health care. Such information is needed at three different levels: global, regional and national (including the local level).

At the global level, one needs primarily to know how many countries have politically committed themselves to developing PHC. The evaluation consists of counting the documents, laws or otherwise, which indicate such commitments.

At the regional level, the task is complicated by the fact that the Regions have adopted their own targets which state specific requirements for the development of PHC. Consequently, one needs to know how these targets have been achieved. At the national level the information needed depends on the national targets and priorities. It should support planning, management and evaluation.

The problem is that the information systems of most countries have not been adapted to take into account the information needs related to the development of PHC.

Could WHO's explicit or implicit policies concerning the information needed for PHC help the Member States to collect the necessary information and to restructure their information systems accordingly?

Health information systems traditionally contain information about: the population, its health status, health risks (including physical and social environment), and the health care system (Nomesko 1985). WHO has specified the information needed for monitoring HFA and PHC as a part of it as follows (WHO 1981b):

(1) Health policy indicators:

- political commitment to health for all;
- resource allocation;
- the degree of equity of distribution of health resources;
- community involvement in attaining health for all;
- organizational framework and managerial process.

(2) Social and economic indicators related to health:

- rate of population increase;
- income distribution;
- gross national product or gross domestic product;
- work conditions;
- adult literary rate;
- housing;
- food availability.

(3) indicators of the provision of health care:

- coverage by primary health care;
- coverage by the referral system;

(4) Health status indicators:

- nutritional status and psychosocial development of children:
- infant mortality rate;
- child mortality rate;
- life expectancy at birth or at other specific ages;
- maternal mortality rate.

An analysis of the current information systems in most Member States against this list would probably reveal that: information related to health policy indicators is not being collected at the national level or the information is purely descriptive; information on most social and economic indicators related to health is being collected but not necessarily used by the health authorities; there is information related to the provision of health services but most of this concerns hospital services; health status indicators may be the strongest component of the current information systems.

An analysis against the four facets of PHC shows, in turn, that the information systems are relatively strong in providing data on PHC activities; they are much poorer in giving a picture of the role of the front line services in the over-all health care system; very little data exist on the implementation of the strategic principles and virtually nothing on the PHC philosophy.

The European Regional Targets (WHO 1984a) further specify the kind of information that is needed to evaluate whether PHC is being implemented or not. They include five targets directly dealing with PHC. The first one requests the establishment of a PHC system supported by secondary and tertiary care; the second specifies that the services should be distributed according to need and that physical, economic and cultural accessibility should support planning, management and evaluation.

The information implications of these targets can be supplemented with those of the blueprint for transforming primary medical care to primary health care and the four facets of PHC. We need information on:

- positive health;
- health needs of the population and attention paid to high risk groups;
- functional ability of the patients;
- distribution of health care resources between primary, secondary and tertiary care;
- distribution of resources between health promotion, prevention, treatment and rehabilitation;
- distribution of health manpower between various categories of health professionals and between generalists and specialists;
- integration of services between different levels of care;
- continuity and comprehensiveness of care;
- organizational settings in which health care providers work;
- extent and nature of intersectorial collaboration;
- extent and nature of community participation;
- extent and nature of lay care;
- physical, social and cultural accessibility of care;
- social acceptability of care; and
- use of technology within different sectors of care.

DIFFICULTIES AND CHALLENGES

The provision of such information is a tall order - difficult but challenging.

Difficulties

In 1984, the European Member States made the first valiant attempt to assess their achievements with regard to HFA using the proposed regional indicators. The results were reported to the Regional Committee in 1985 (WHO 1985). They revealed several difficulties.

The report is replete with statements such as: "The lack of data to measure equity (or inequity) among countries ..."; lifestyle indicators are not easy to measure"; "information on tobacco consumption is not systematically collected"; "the national and regional data [on drugs] are scanty and not easily comparable"; "data patterns on recreation and exercise are generally not available and information on trends is equally scarce"; "only ten countries provided information on the distribution of the health expenditure between local health care and other levels of care"; "the definition of "local health care" varied considerably"; the available data are rarely broken down between primary health care and other services"; "caution must be exercised because of the difficulty of obtaining precise and comparable definitions of what is covered by the term "hospital beds"..."; and "the assessments [of trends in health care system] have to be based mainly on non-quantitative indicators and general descriptive texts".

The difficulties can be grouped under some main headings: lack of data; lack of quantification; poor and varying definitions; inadequate data collection mechanisms; political reluctance to collect data on controversial topics; use of lack of data as an excuse for delaying decisions; lack of baseline data for establishing trends; difficulties in using data collected for other sectors; incompatibility of information systems developed for different parts of the health care system; unclear division of labour and responsibility between institutions charged with collecting the data; insufficient collaboration and coordination between such institutions; neglect of management needs in the analysis and publication of data; neglect of the need to analyze and aggregate the data differently for different levels of the health care system and different users of the information; and lacking specification of the use to be made of the collected data.

These problems are likely to hit worst the level where information about PHC would be needed most - the local level.

All these deficiencies have to be addressed when developing an information system for PHC. The evaluation report particularly highlighted the need for: improvement of the quality of data on disease incidence; promotion of the use of the standard classification of impairments, disabilities and handicaps; classification and standardization of work-related disorders; more precise definition of community involvement and finding ways of measuring both its extent and its effects; and a review of nutritional policy and indicators (WHO 1985)

Challenges

It is admittedly difficult to develop - let alone quantify - suitable indicators for many PHC goals, such as political commitment, community participation, closeness to the population, relevance to the needs, use of appropriate technology and social acceptability. Information specialists have a tendency to look askance at qualitative indicators as their validity, reliability, sensitivity, specificity, i.e. the usual characteristics one would expect from a statistical indicator are impossible to ascertain. The qualitative nature of many PHC indicators can even be evoked to delay purposively action.

In spite of the difficulties, there are encouraging signs that many Member States are willing to face the challenge. One indication is that all Member States returned the evaluation questionnaire and had done their best to provide all the requested information. All the 65 essential regional indicators or groups of indicators were covered by one or more countries, but there was great variation in coverage and for some indicators there was not sufficient information to give a regional picture.

Several countries stressed the importance of timely and relevant information for health management. At least two countries had shaped their own health information systems in accordance with the suggested regional indicators. Some countries have established information units to provide systematic and analytical information on health services, to conduct monitoring surveys, and to evaluate the development, implementation, relevance, efficiency and cost-effectiveness of such programmes. In many countries, measures are being taken to develop national data banks on health and social services (WHO 1985).

It is, however, not enough to provide the decision-makers, planners, administrators and health care providers with appropriate information. Such information is also intended to stimulate public awareness of, and participation in, health problems and their solutions. Consequently, communication with the public is essential if there is to be more awareness and political support. The public not only needs greater access to health information but also needs that information in a form it can use.

LITERATURE

World Health Organization, Geneva (1977) Thirtieth World Health Assembly, Resolution 30.43

World Health Organization (1978) Health for All Series No. 1, Primary Health Care

Vuori, H (1982) Primary Health Care in Industrialized countries. J Royal College of General Practitioners 72: 729-735

Vuori, H (1984a) General Practitioners: Allies or Enemies of Primary Health Care. Scand J Prim Health Care 2 57-61

Vuori, H (1984b) Primary Health Care in Europe - Problems and Solutions. Community Medicine 6: 221-231

McKeown, T (1976) The role of medicine. Dream, Mirage or Nemesis? The Nuffield Provincial Hospital Trust, London

Vuori, H (1980) Development and Information needs of Primary Health Care in Europe. In the Computer in the Doctor's Office. Reinhoff, A and Abrams M E (eds.) North Holland, Amsterdam

The Swedish Ministry of Health and Social Affairs (1981) Primary Health Care Today, Some International Comparisons, Stockholm, Sweden

Vuori, H (1984c) Information Needs of Primary Health Care. In Third International Conference on System Science in Health Care, van Eimeren, W, Engelbrecht, R and Flagle, Ch.D (eds.)

Vuori, H (1985) The role of the Schools of Public Health in the Development of Primary Health Care. Health Policy, 4: 221-230, Eslevier

World Health Organization, Geneva (1981). Health for All Series no. 3Global Strategy for Health for All by the Year 2000

World Health Organization, Geneva (1981) Health for All Series No. 4. Development of Indicators for Monitoring Progress Towards Health for All by the Year 2000

World Health Organization Regional Office for Europe, Copenhagen (1980) Regional Strategy for Obtaining Health for All by the Year 2000

World Health Organization Regional Office for Europe, Copenhagen (1984a) Regional Targets in Support of the Regional Strategy for Health for All

World Health Organization Regional Office for Europe, Copenhagen (1984b) Report on the Thirty-Fourth Session of the Regional Committee for Europe

World Health Organization Regional Office for Europe, Copenhagen (1985) Regional Evaluation

Nordisk Medicinal-Statistisk Kommitté (NOMESKO) (1985) Datorstödda informationssystem inom primärvarden i Norden, Helsingfors

PRIMARY HEALTH CARE IN CANADA - A REVIEW OF SYSTEMS

Richard MacLachlan, Associate Professor, Department of Family Medicine, Dalhousie University, Halifax, Canada

Primary health care in Canada is provided in most instances by physicians. Regional responsibility for health care coupled with fee-for-service government sponsored medical insurance creates an accounting and data processing task ideally suited to computerization. Other uses of the systems are presented and anticipated directions for future growth are outlined.

Primary health care delivery in Canada has been profoundly affected by two related factors--our geography and our political evolution. Canada has the second largest land mass of any country in the world yet has one of the smaller populations in countries of the developed western world with uneven distribution. Thus, access to services varies greatly from location to location within the country. As well, our colonization by European powers and eventual evolution into an independent Commonwealth country resulted in many traditional governmental powers being based regionally, or provincially. Health and education are two of the most important in this regard.

Primary health care is provided in first instance in almost all parts of Canada by physicians, with the notable exceptions being:

(1) Well child care, including immunizations, which is frequently provided by provincial health nurses.

(2) Out-post health care in the far north where specially trained nurses provide the primary care, with physician back-up.

(3) Community health centres where nurse practitioners provide some primary care.

(4) Special services such as chiropractic, podiatry, chiropody, and in some instances physiotherapy; however, these services are often not covered by health care insurance unless the patient is referred by a physician.

(5) Pharmacists or chemists who provide counselling about minor ailments and recommendations about nonprescription drug therapy.

Primary Care Medical Practice

In 1982, Canada's population was approaching 25 million and we had 44,216 physicians licenced for practice. If we look at data from a nationwide physician survey that year[1] which had an 87% response rate (Table 1), we are able to review the profile of those.

Since 1968, we have had special training programs for physicians wishing to work in family practice. These programs are not yet compulsory for practitioners entering general primary care but there is a strong movement in this regard in many parts of the country. For the purposes of this paper, I am grouping together general practitioners and family physicians, and will address them as the former.

I have found it impossible to get accurate information on the extent to which specialists in for example paediatrics, obstetrics, and internal medicine provide primary care. In consultation with others across the country, I would venture an upper estimate of 5 - 10% in these specialties. You can see from Table 1 that there is approximately one provider of primary medical care for every 1,597 persons.

Table 1

Physicians in Primary Health Care in Canada - 1982

12,276*	General Practice/Family Practice
491*	Emergency Medicine
450*	Primary Care Specialties **
2,439*	Other ***
15,656*	Total

*: of the 38,653 respondents (87.4% of licensed physicians)

**: estimate based on 10% of Paediatrics, Obstetrics/Gynecology and Internal Medicine

***: 2,411 non-specialist respondents did not appropriately answer the question "Did general or family best describe their practice"?. It is estimated that 2/3 of these are in GP/FP.

Adapted from Woodward[1]

Primary care physicians represent 41% of all physicians in the country with some fluctuations from province to province; in the far north, they represent nearly 3/4's of all physicians.[1] Also noteworthy is the fact that over 80% of physicians licenced in 1982 were males. With women representing 30% to in excess of 50% of medical school admissions, this is expected to change dramatically over the next decade.

As mentioned earlier, our geography plays a major factor in access to primary care. One-third of the population resides in centres of less than 10,000 persons;[2] these centres have only 19% of the general practitioners. As a result, individual patients may have to go a significant distance to get care, and some rural physicians have quite large populations to serve.

The 1982 survey concluded that 48 hours per week were spent on average in direct patient care by general practitioners, excluding time "on-call". This was quite close to the comparable figures for specialists. The majority of the time spent in patient care by general practitioners is in ambulatory care; I don't have hard data on this but would estimate that it would range from 60% for a general practitioner with a busy hospital and obstetrical practice to nearly 100% for some general practitioners practising near large teaching hospitals in urban centres.

The vast majority of Canadian general practitioners form some group arrangements. These range from a series of solo practices with individual physicians covering each other's practices after hours to the shared facilities of a group practice, to a partnership with formal economic interactions and commitments. The latter two arrangements have not been as popular in Canada as in our close neighbour to the south and solo practice with off-hours shared coverage has remained very strong and viable in Canada.

The typical Canadian general practitioner has between 1,000 - 2,000 patients; these patients consult the physician 4 - 5 times annually on average, with fluctuations depending on the age structure of the practice and the availability of other services.

Health Care Expenditures

If we are to consider expenditures in health care in Canada, three measures are perhaps most useful for comparison:

(1) 7.8% of the gross national product was directed towards health care in 1981.[3]

(2) This represented an estimated $586 Canadian per capita ($450 US at 1985 conversion rate).[4]

(3) The average physician income after expenses but before taxes in 1982 was $75,000 ($57,700 U.S.).[5]

Remuneration of physicians in Canada for primary health care is based on two principles:

(1) A universal health insurance available to all residents of the country.

(2) A fee-for-service based system of payments to physicians and other providers with some exceptions.

Government-sponsored health insurance for medical and hospital services has gradually extended over the last 28 years to the point where only a very small percentage of funding for medical services in Canada came from private sources in 1983. The Canada Health Act of 1984 was an attempt by the federal government to remove all private funding of medical services through user fees and extra billing by physicians beyond the agreed-upon fees-for-services, and the disparity among provinces over premiums charged for health insurange. The principles of universality, comprehensiveness, accessibility, portability, and public administration were declared as cardinal to the continued effectiveness of the insurance;[6] at this time there are still ongoing disagreements between the different levels of government in some provinces. As health care is a provincial responsibility, the federal governments main lever has been the introduction of financial penalties for non-conforming provinces.[7]

Community Health Centres

There are some notable exceptions to the model I have described thus far; these represent community health centres (C.H.C.). There are many descriptions and definitions of what a C.H.C. is; using a basic one[8] (Figure 1), there were 146 of these in Canada in 1981, and there are now just under 200.

Figure 1

Community Health Centres

- A Board of Directors who are not physicians at the centre
- At least one professional who is not a physician plus at least one physician on staff
- Physicians are remunerated on other than fee-for-service basis.

From Health Link, 1982

Many of these centres have received funding on a capitation basis from the provincial medical insurance plan; this gives them a fixed amount per person per year in some cases corrected for such factors as age. The Board of the C.H.C. is then free to allocate these funds according to how they best feel is appropriate to provide effective primary care for their patients. In many cases non-physicians are employed to provide primary care and, in fact, C.H.C.'s effectively provide the only way in which a nurse-practitioner can provide primary care in a community setting.

A recent innovation has been to monitor the utilization of hospital services by patients registered with a C.H.C. A percentage of any savings perceived in comparing their utilization with that of the general population is returned to the C.H.C. and is an incentive to be cost-conscious and orient themselves towards disease prevention. In one large industrial urban centre in Ontario, Sault St. Marie, approximately half of the population is registered with community health centres. While C.H.C.'s provide care for only a very small percentage of Canadians, they do represent an alternate model of primary care delivery that is receiving careful scrutiny and cautious support in at least three provinces, as one possible avenue to control health care costs while not eliminating services.

Surveillance

Surveillance of primary health care services is provided at two levels. The quality of care delivered is monitored by the medical licensing bodies and by institutions such as hospitals and nursing homes; this represents in effect peer review. There is at present some movement from a complaint-based review process to a prospective audit-based program whereby actual patient records would be reviewed and compared with agreed-upon minimal standards.[9] The other form of review is a more traditional audit by the medical insurance bodies and taxation departments, using largely sampling techniques to ensure that services charged for were in fact provided, and that funding received was reported as income.

Accounting and Office Management

The fee-for-service system of remuneration for physicians creates very specific requirements for accounting. Figure 2 outlines the most common pieces of data required by the provincial medicare plans in Canada. This information is submitted on forms or computer cards which are read by personnel and key punched, or by optical character readers. The diagnoses are coded either manually or electronically usually to some variant of ICD-9.

Figure 2

Accounting Requirements - Fee-for-service Medical Insurance

Demographic:	Name, Address, Birthdate, Identification Number
Diagnostic:	Diagnosis (Free-text or code)
Procedural:	Service provided (when, where, and what - usually code)
Economic:	Fee claimed

This has been the logical point of entry for many physicians to consider using a computer in their office. These data handling tasks are routine, repetitive, and are at high risk for human error in transcription with major economic implications. As well, the health insurers have a massive data handling task, far greater than capitation-based systems, with the main input of data requiring human translation, and clearly a mechanism which reduces the data handling time and costs, and increases reliability is of interest.

The accounting and billing benefits of computer use in primary care practice have been a major boost to the introduction of systems, and savings through improved accounting practices have offset or justified the costs involved. There are, however, many other tasks which computers handle in primary care practices in Canada. (Figure 3) With accurate demographic data in each patient file, it has been relatively straightforward to create appointment schedules, recall and chronic problem lists, and even patient profiles of diagnoses and medications. Only a small number of systems have moved into computerization of medical record, faced with the obvious problems of handling large amounts of free-text information and the difficulties posed in retrieval of particular pieces of information at a later date.

Figure 3

Computer Usage in General Practice - Tasks

- Demographic
- Billing
- Other administrative, eg. appointments
- Word Processing
- Research
- Recall, Chronic Problems
- Patient profile (Problems, Medications)
- Periodic Health Maintenance
- Partial (Full Medical Record)
- Communication (Data Bases, Institutions...)

Communication with existing data bases has been the subject of an interesting research project this last year in which 15 medical practices across the country were provided with a video display telephone that allowed them to call up data bases on medical subject headings, drug toxicology, and many others, and print abstracts in their office. The results of this study will be available early in 1986.

Finally, research projects, have been greatly facilitated with the ability of general practitioners to extract information from their demographic, diagnostic, and procedural data using a report-generating program. All of this data was previously being processed manually with no easy means of retrieval; research is thus possible for some questions with little or no extra time commitments.

Penetration of Computers into Primary Care

If we consider now the penetration of computers into Canadian primary care practices, the information available and the estimated penetration varies tremendously from province to province. I received responses to my request for information from 8 of the 10 provinces and 2 territories, and the following comments are based on those responses:

(1) All provinces have some utilization of computers by primary care physicians; this ranges from one solo general practitioner in one province, to another province where 2/3's of all claims for all services (including laboratory) are submitted on magnetic tape,

(2) The differing provincial requirements for billing submissions have resulted in software development being limited to regional use.

(3) Critical factors in system development in each province would appear to be

    i.) The willingness/ability of the provincial medicare body to accept machine readable submissions.

    ii.) The number of practising physicians.

(4) The most common form of submission to medicare is by magnetic tape; the development of private service bureaus has allowed individuals with personal computers to make submissions on diskettes with subsequent translation to magnetic tape. One province, Ontario, has allowed physicians to submit billings on 5¼" diskettes since May, 1984, and approximately 16% of the potential users are now submitting in this manner.

(5) Involvement of professional organizations has varied greatly from province to province, ranging from little or no activity due to small numbers and little demand, to major involvement in software development, hardware selection, and package promotion.

Problems

Introduction of computer systems into primary care practices has not happened without significant problems developing. As described earlier, differing regional requirements and the need for accreditation to allowing billing of medicare insurers has restricted nation-wide program development. This coupled with the rapidly changing technology of computer hardware and software, and inappropriate expectations by physicians as to the capabilities of both has resulted in many systems, particularly those more than 4 years old, collecting dust in the corner.

With the rapid expansion of data banks containing personal information, the issues of privacy controls - the protection of the confidentiality of the patient's medical information, has become an important issue. One can easily visualize the "benefits" as measured by more efficient patient care of a computer network linking the patient's primary care physician, their pharmacist or chemist, their hospital and laboratory, and other health care providers. Yet without extremely comprehensive security checks in the system, patient confidentiality could potentially vanish.

Trends in usage

Looking to the next decade of primary care computer systems in Canada, I see three areas of major development:

(1) Increasing linkage of primary care providers with other parts of the health care system—hospitals, chemists, other providers.

(2) Major advances in the way we handle free-text medical information from medical records.

(3) Computer-aided diagnosis, management, and patient education.

I see the result of this being major improvements in the organization and delivery of primary health care. We must ensure, however, that this is not at the expense of the patient-physician relationship.

I would like to express my thanks to Helen Robson and other members of the Department of Medical Economics, Canadian Medical Association for their generous assistance in the preparation of this paper.

References

1. Woodward C, Adams O: *Physician resource databank: numbers, distribution and activities of Canada's physicians.* Can Med Assoc J 1985; 132:1,175 - 1,188

2. Statistics Canada

3. *Preserving Universal Medicare.* Minister of Supply and Services Canada 1983; H21-92/1983, p 13

4. ibid, p 14

5. *Physicians' Management Manuals.* MacLean-Hunter. February 1985 p 14

6. *Preserving Universal Medicare.* Minister of Supply and Services Canada 1983; H21-92/1983 p 9

7. *Intercom.* Manitoba Medical Association 1985; 105:1

8. *Health Link.* Ontario Department of Health 1982; 2:1

9. McAuley RG, Henderson HW: *Results of the Peer Assessment Program of the College of Physicians and Surgeons of Ontario.* Can Med Assoc J. 1984; 131:557 -561.

AN OVERVIEW OF PRIMARY HEALTH CARE IN SOUTH AFRICA AND THE EFFECT OF MEDICAL AID INSURANCE ON PRIVATE PRACTITIONERS

Don Struthers

Director, Practice Management Plans (Pty) Ltd.,
P.O. Box 5780, Johannesburg, 2000, Republic of South Africa.

INTRODUCTION

South Africa is a land of extreme contrasts. Besides vast differences in the ethnic origins, traditions, cultural, economic and political backgrounds making it such a complex society, the population is also quite unevenly distributed across a wide divergence of rural, urban and metropolitan areas.

It is both a developing and an industrialised country at the same time. A strange - and probably unique - mix of First and Third Worlds, together with varying stages of advancement at all levels in between.

Although there is no national health programme in operation, a multiplicity of modern amenities and facilities are provided for the care and well-being of the different race groups throughout the land. At least 75 percent of the population - mainly Blacks, Coloureds, Indians and Whites who are not covered by medical aid insurance - receive either free or subsidised medical services rendered by government agencies.

General practitioners and specialists in all categories cater for an estimated 25 percent of private patients who are charged on a fee for service basis. The majority of this segment are Whites, but an increasing number of the other population groups are now also becoming members of pre-paid medical insurance schemes which provide a minimum range of benefits in terms of statutory legislation. It is not compulsory for private practitioners to render services in accordance with the fee structure and specific administrative procedures laid down by the Medical Schemes Act and they are, therefore, free to deal with their patients differently according to each particular set of circumstances.

Primary health services in the developing or "deep rural" areas, where upwards of 45 percent of the Black indigineous people are situated, are usually provided by regional and local authorities. These may typically include a referral hospital, a district hospital with surrounding clinics and mobile units visiting remote points where practical. Here the extended role of suitably qualified, registered nurses plays a vital role in bringing curative, promotive and preventive care to the community. The effectiveness of such facilities varies quite dramatically from one region to another, depending on many variable factors, and remains a highly controversial subject both locally and abroad.

A further sharp contrast to the advanced Western medical care centred around the developed areas is found in the support of traditional healers, or so-called "witch doctors", by a fairly large number of the Black population. Tribal medicine, with its aura of the supernatural, is part of their early culture and even today is by no means restricted to the far outlying rural areas.

Apart from these widely divergent social and geographic conditions, both the public and private sectors are involved in the delivery of varying levels of primary health care services, and it is against this somewhat intricate background, that the analysis of the present environment in South Africa should be approached.

The use of computers in primary care at present is almost exclusively confined to patient accounting and similar financial control systems for private practitioners. These are provided by a wide range of service organisations, microcomputer vendors and software houses. Increasing awareness, however, shows that there is both interest and need for further development across a broad spectrum of clinical applications.

THE STRUCTURE OF PRIMARY HEALTH CARE IN SOUTH AFRICA

Primary care in terms of the South African situation can be divided into two main streams, general practice in its various forms and institutionally based PHC. The latter embraces many patterns of practice, from the outpatient department of a general hospital, right through all the varieties of community oriented services to the smallest clinic. It is also true that many practitioners are involved in several different aspects of medical care. There are those who are also part-time medical officers of health or who do sessional duty at a hospital in the out-patient or casualty department. Others serve as honorary medical officers to institutions like old-age homes and sports clubs.

This description does not take into account the many other agencies, including large employer groups and voluntary organisations, outside the medical profession that are involved in health care for the community of South Africa (Nel 1984).

Some answers to the question of who delivers primary care, where and when are provided in the following outline of the different roles undertaken by the public and private sectors.

The Public Sector

The organisation of health services at government level agrees significantly with the general administration of the country, and is the responsibility of three agencies, namely the Central Government, the four Provincial Administrations and some 400 Local Authorities. The Health Act of 1977 established a National Health Policy Council and a Health Matters Advisory Committee to co-ordinate all health services rendered by these three tiers of government, which are summarised as follows.

The Department of Health and Welfare

In terms of current legislation, community health is the responsibility of the Department of Health and Welfare with its head office in Pretoria, working through decentralised regional offices staffed by medical and ancillary members of the health-care team (South Africa 1985).
Broad functions of the Department include the maintenance of health chemistry and other laboratory services, provision of research institutions, promotion of family planning services, environmental and medico-legal services, prevention of disease and the provision of all facilities necessary for the promotion of health. It is specifically

responsible for the control over mental institutions and hospitals for tuberculosis patients and lepers, and ensures that the health services provided by local authorities are properly managed.

The Department also provides district nursing, detached out-patient and other primary care services in certain areas.

Provincial Administrations

All hospital facilities and auxiliary services required within the scope of curative health care are provided by the four provincial administrations. In addition they are responsible for out-patient and casualty facilities, maternity hospitals and services, and the treatment of acute mental disorders. Detached clinics with district nurses delivering primary health care to local communities are well established in several areas.

Most large general hospitals, including the teaching hospitals of medical schools are administered by the provinces. These are situated in cities, towns and larger centres, forming a network which covers the entire country apart from the Black national states. Facilities are provided for the full range of the most sophisticated up-to-date procedures, including organ transplants, all fields of major surgery, dialysis and radiation therapy. In cases where specialised treatment of any category is not available in smaller outlying clinics, patients are transferred to these larger hospitals by provincial ambulances (South Africa 1985).

The Day Hospitals Organisation

The Day Hospitals Organisation was started in the Cape Peninsula in 1969 to provide a primary health care service in the community for those people in the lower income group not covered by medical insurance. These units equate more with community health centres than with specialised day hospitals. Here the family practitioner has become the leader of a modern health team, consisting of other practitioners, nursing personnel, district sisters, midwives, social workers, physiotherapists, radiographers and pharmacists.

Patients attending day hospitals or visited at home can be placed into five categories: those with common episodic illness requiring diagnosis, treatment and management; those with serious disease or trauma requiring immediate emergency care or referral; those with long-term or progressive illness requiring management and periodic evaluation; those requiring after-care and rehabilitation after discharge from a hospital; and the low risk obstetric patient (Smith 1981).

Local Authorities

Urban and rural local authorities are responsible for all community and environmental services in their areas of jurisdiction. The health services are subsidised by the central Government, which exercises the necessary control by means of legislation, financial assistance as well as systematic inspections.

Their comprehensive range of personal services include those for ante and post-natal care, family planning, care for the aged, child health services, health visits at home and domiciliary midwifery services where they are not supplied by hospitals.

Community Involvement in terms of The Health Act

In keeping with the modern accepted concept that the community should participate in health matters, it is one of the aims of the Health Act of 1977 to involve the community in selective priority determination and rendition of supplementary services. This can take place either on an organised or on an ad-hoc basis, with special recognition of the role of all responsible voluntary organisations (Guide to Health Act 1977).

The Private Sector

There are various concepts of primary care and general practice in South Africa. The South African Medical and Dental Council has held that a general practitioner is a doctor who is not on the specialist register. Public opinion, and that of many doctors, still holds that a general practitioner is a doctor who conducts a non-specialist general practice for which he is in receipt of fees from patients. This definition would exclude, for example, doctors working in rural district hospitals, health centres or other sectors such as district surgeoncies.

The South African Academy designates itself the role of "Family Practice / Primary Care". One of its stated objectives is to "raise the standards of general practice and primary care". Whether the terms general practice, family practice, family medicine and primary care are synonymous and interchangeable, or constitute separate components of some undefined discipline seeking to specialise in its own generality may require clarification (Spencer 1984).

It is, however, necessary to establish a base line for discussions on how computers are being applied in the primary care environment of South Africa. For the purpose of this Conference's analysis and systems comparison, attention has been focused around the private general practitioner described in the first paragraph above, more especially since this is the main area in which computers are currently being used.

Personnel

The following medical personnel were registered with their respective Council's or Board's at the end of each year shown.

Category	1983	1984
Medical Practitioners	18 109	19 294
Dentists	3 069	3 262
Specialists (Medical)	4 350	4 833
Specialists (Dental)	192	209
Interns	1 077	1 075
Supplementary Health Personnel	16 789	18 824
Medical Students	4 441	6 271
Dental Students	1 055	992
Registered Nurses, including Midwives	60 941	*
Enrolled Nurses	19 986	*
Enrolled Nursing Assistants	37 571	*
Pharmacists	6 452	6 815
Trainee Pharmacists	402	480
Supplementary Health Students	*	5 931

* Figures not available
Source: South Africa Foundation 1986 Information Digest

It is estimated that approximately half of the registered medical practitioners are employed in various categories by the public sector and that the other half are engaged in different structures of private practice. Specialists are not really active in primary care, since having qualified and registered as such with the S.A. Medical and Dental Council, their first contact with private patients should only be through referral by a general practitioner. This is, however, somewhat of a controversial issue in a number of circles.

Total Health Expenditure

More recent figures are not available, but according to Retief (1984), the estimated total expenditure of the public and private sectors on "health" in South Africa during 1980 was R2 725 million or 4,6 percent of the Gross National Product. The latter figure lies between the 2 to 3 percent spent in developing countries and the 5 to 6 percent spent in developed countries, as does the per capita expenditure which, in 1980, was R52.

State Budget

Details of the State budget in respect of health and welfare promotion for 1984/5 are as follows (Dept. Health Annual Report, 1984):

Programmes and Objectives	Rands
Administration	18 653 000
Infectious, Communicable and Other Diseases	80 433 000
Mental Health	141 023 000
Medical Care	86 964 000
Health Protection	32 057 000
Associated and Auxiliary Services	115 510 000
Internal Charges	25 150 000
Welfare Promotion	554 804 000

Private Practitioner's Income

The Bureau of Financial Analysis (1984) attached to the University of Pretoria has published the results of a survey into private general practice which was commissioned by the National General Practitioners Group of the Medical Association of South Africa. Questionnaires were sent to 4 200 doctors in private practice and a final sample of 11,8 percent was used to arrive at the following gross and net income profile of an "average" general practitioner in South Africa as at 28 February, 1983.

Professional Fees	R75 064
Part-time Appointments	3 993
Other Income	2 460
Total Gross Income	R81 518
Less Expenses	42 404
Net Income	R39 113

The Bureau went further in its analysis and produced the following comparison between the averages of the best twenty and the worst twenty returns which it received:

Details	Best 20	Worst 20
Total Income	R153 623	R47 520
Less Expenses	59 589	35 639
Net Income	R 94 034	R11 880

There are naturally many private practitioners' income profiles which would vary quite significantly with those reflected in the Bureau's findings. Determining factors would include the geographic situation of the practice, the patient profile and nature of services rendered, fees charged according to medical aid or private rates, solo, associate or partnership structure, hours worked, administrative and auxiliary personnel, management style, and many more.

Doctors in the full-time employment of the public sector are paid according to a fixed salary scale which may include certain special allowances. Their annual income ranges from about R30 000 upwards, depending on their qualifications and the nature of duties performed.

THE POPULATION

One of the most marked characteristics of the South African population is its heterogenity. The many sub-sections are usually classified into four main groups, each with its own contrasting ethnic origins, traditions, cultures and stages of socio-economic development. The 1985 preliminary census results, without adjustments for undercount are as follows:

Category	millions
Blacks	15 242 828
Coloureds	2 825 094
Indians	793 978
Whites	4 576 690
Total Population RSA	23 438 590

Structure of the Peoples

The greater part of the White population is either English or Afrikaans speaking. Afrikaans derives from the Dutch language introduced by settlers in the seventeenth century. The major English settlement took place in 1820. English and Afrikaans are both official languages of the country.

The Coloureds are a people of mixed descent, with White, Black, Malay and Khoisan ancestors. The Indian community is descended mainly from labourers brought to work on the Natal sugar plantations during the nineteenth century.

The Black peoples are made up of four main linguistic groupings, the Nguni, the Sotho, the Venda and the Shangaan-Tsonga, with a number of sub-divisions in each group. The major Nguni languages are Zulu, Xhosa, Swazi and Ndebele; the major Sotho languages are Southern Sotho, North Sotho (Pedi) and Tswana.

Catchment Areas

South Africa is approximately 1 120 000 square km in extent, over five times the size of Britain and approximately equal to the combined area of West Germany, France, Italy, the Netherlands and Belgium. It is divided into four provinces, namely the Transvaal, Orange Free State, Natal and the Cape Province.

Legislation initiated in 1959 has lead to the creation of independent national states in which Blacks exercise political rights and control over their own affairs. There are ten such states established on ethnic principles and four have been granted independence status.

The most thickly populated parts of the country are the four major industrial areas, the Pretoria-Witwatersrand-Vereeniging (PWV) area, the Durban-Pinetown-Pietermaritzburg area, the south-western Cape and the Port Elizabeth-Uitenhage area. More than a third of the total population lives in these four regions, accounting for 80 percent of the total urban population, although the four areas together constitute only 4 percent of the total geographic area.

80 percent of the Indians live in Natal and nearly 90 percent of the Coloureds in the Cape Province. Overall population density is 18 per square km compared with 24 in the United States, 97 in France and 228 in the United Kingdom (South Africa 1985).

The ten National States comprise 13,12 percent of the total area of South Africa. Their populations are as follows:

Independent National States	millions
Transkei	2 912 408
Bophuthatswana	1 667 478
Venda	381 891
Ciskei	903 681
Total	5 865 458
Self-governing States	
Gazankulu	580 952
KaNgwane	377 898
KwaNdebele	176 727
KwaZulu	3 866 273
Lebowa	2 046 479
QwaQwa	178 124
Total	7 226 453
Grand Total	13 091 911

Source: SA Institute of Race Relations Survey 1984

Morbidity Statistics

Benatar and Saven (1985) report that in 1971, 5 544 patients were admitted to the 261 Department of Medicine beds at Groote Schuur Hospital. During 1982, 8 005 were admitted although the number of beds remained essentially unchanged. Whites constituted 54,7 percent of all admissions in 1971 and 39,9 percent in 1982. The overall mortality rate fell from 14,9 percent in 1971 to 9,6 percent in 1982, and the respective autopsy rates from 25,9 percent to 18,2 percent.

Patterns of morbidity observed in the various population groups differed greatly and changed over the period studied. Comparisons between the hospital patients and national mortality patterns showed great parallels within each population group and major differences between the different groups - those in Whites closely resemble patterns in industrialised countries, whereas for the patients of mixed race and Black patients they more closely approximate those in developing countries.

The overall distribution of diagnoses and percentages in the major ICD categories (*) for 1971 and 1982 are as follows:

Disease Category	1971 - percent	- 1982
Infectious and parasitic diseases	6,3 (000-136)	7,4 (001-139)
Neoplasms	5,7 (140-239)	5,9 (140-239)
Endocrine / nutritional / metabolic disorders	9,5 (240-279)	11,2 (240-279)
Diseases of the blood and blood forming organs	3,0 (280-289)	3,9 (280-289)
Mental disorders	3,4 (290-315)	2,7 (290-319)
Disease of nervous system and sensory organs	2,9 (320-389)	4,2 (320-389)
Diseases of circulatory system	44,4 (390-458)	42,8 (390-459)
Diseases of respiratory system	12,6 (460-519)	9,8 (460-519)
Diseases of digestive system	8,9 (520-577)	9,9 (520-577)
Musculoskeletal system and connective tissue	3,3 (710-738)	2,6 (710-739)
Total No. of patients	5 544	8 005
Total No. of diagnosis	9 308	15 424
Diagnosis / patient	1,7	1,9

* ICD numbers (for 1971 from the 8th revision and for 1982 from the 9th revision) given in parenthesis.

Mobility of Choice, Access and Treatment Periods

Private patients and members of medical aid societies have complete freedom of choice with easy access to all facilities in the major centres. Treatment periods as such are not prescribed by any particular legislation and would necessarily depend on the nature of each condition. Medical schemes may, however, impose benefit restrictions in some cases.

STRUCTURE OF PRIVATE PRACTICES

The survey undertaken by the Bureau of Financial Analysis (1984) also examined several aspects relating to the overall structure of private general practice in South Africa. Although the "average" profile will again vary quite dramatically according to different circumstances, an interesting pattern is established from the results of its findings as summarised below:

Solo Practice and Group Partnerships

Inspite of there being few respondents in the larger categories, the following percentage breakdown as to the number of doctors in solo practice and group partnerships is considered to be representative:

Number of Partners	Percentage
Solo Practice	71,3
Two Partners	11,6
Three Partners	6,3
Four Partners	6,9
Five Partners	2,6
Six Partners	1,0
Seven Partners	,3

Age Distribution

Less than 30 years	5,5
31 to 40 years	42,0
41 to 50 years	23,4
51 to 60 years	18,2
Over 60 years	10,9

The report does not indicate how many of the solo practitioners work together in association as opposed to being in a formal partnership. It should also be noted that whilst mixed professionals are found in out-patient departments at provincial hospitals and clinics administered by the public sector, general practitioners and specialists in private practice may not share consulting rooms with common facilities.

General Information According to Age Category

Respondents to the survey were also asked to submit certain general information which was analysed according to their age category:

	Age in Years				
Details	- 30	31-40	41-50	51-60	+ 60
Years in Practice	2,48	7,83	15,39	27,40	38,19
Years in Current Practice	2,33	5,97	11,03	20,56	32,24
Days of Absence for					
Vacation	33	28	25	22	25
Sickness	1	2	1	5	7
Congresses / Study	5	4	4	3	4

Activity and Time Analysis

One of the most interesting aspects of the Bureau's Report is the analysis of the "average" private general practitioner's activities during a typical four week period, and how much time is allocated to the different functions which he performs. The findings show that some 75 hours per week are spent in the practice, with slightly more than 40 hours (53 percent) being devoted to consultations in respect of approximately 150 patients. This works out to an average of flow of 3,8 patients per hour or 15,8 minutes per consultation.

The balance of time was split between visits, hospital activities, practice administration, continuing education, research, part-time work and other outside interests.

Distribution of Private Practitioners

Private practitioners tend to be concentrated in and around the major developed areas in much the same proportion as the distribution of the population. The doctor / patient ratio for the country as a whole is approximately 1:1600, but because of the maldistribution, it is far more favourable in the affluent centres than in the deep rural districts.

REMUNERATION

Private practitioners in South Africa have the choice to render services according to a Guide established by the Medical Association, generally referred to as "private fees", or a statutory tarriff, known as the "scale of benefits", which is determined by consultation between the Medical Association and the Representative Association of Medical Schemes in terms of the Medical Schemes Act. At present there is a sharp disparity between the comparative fees of R18,90 and R9,50 for a normal consultation, which is due to a fairly recent increase suggested by the MASA which is expected to be followed by a reasonable adjustment in the medical benefit rate during January, 1986.

Medical Aid Schemes

Approximately 25 percent of the population are covered by some form of medical aid insurance. Most employers provide this as a fringe benefit for eligible personnel and usually contribute at least 50 percent towards the subscriptions, which are determined according to the member's income and number of dependants.

The schemes are administered by employer groups, professional societies and private enterprise, subject to the control of a Central Council established in terms of the Medical Schemes Act. At the end of December, 1984, there were 217 registered schemes and a further 51 which were exempted by virtue of industrial labour agreements.

Prior to December, 1984, private practitioners had a choice of being either "contracted-in" or "contracted-out" on a blanket basis insofar as their dealings with members of registered medical aid schemes were concerned. Those who elected to be contracted-in were then obliged to render their services to all such members according to the statutory tariff and also to follow certain prescribed administrative procedures regarding both the rendition and collection of their accounts.

The legislation has since been amended and practitioners may now decide whether to charge private or medical aid rates according to each individual set of circumstances. However, only fully specified accounts for services rendered in accordance with the scale of benefits are paid by the medical schemes directly to the practice. In all other cases patients are personally responsible for payment of their own accounts and for claiming a re-imbursement based on the scale of benefits and the rules of their own particular scheme.

Medical Benefit Societies

There are also several medical benefit societies administered by very large employer groups, such as the mining industry, which do not allow their members freedom of choice. Under this system doctors are employed on either a fixed salary or a per capita basis to cater for an estimated optimum of 500 members or family units.

Benefits Paid by Medical Aid Schemes

Benefits paid out by registered medical schemes for services rendered to their members and dependants by private general practitioners during the year ended 31 December, 1984, amounted to R136 497 017. Further sums of R20 121 539 and R20 555 802 were paid out by medical benefit schemes and exempted schemes, constituting a grand total of R177 174 358, which represented 17,2 percent of the medical aid movement's total benefit payout for that year. Of the balance, 19,9 percent was paid in respect of specialist services, 12,8 percent for dental services, 18,0 percent for hospitalisation, 25,8 percent for medicine and 6,3 percent for other benefits (Registrar of Medical Schemes 1984).

Surveillance and Peer Review

A Cost Awareness / Peer Review Committee was formed by the Medical Association of South Africa during 1982. Its terms of reference were to enhance awareness among doctors of the cost of medical care they render and to establish a peer review programme. Education plays a major role in each of these functions and the more serious allegations of malpractice are referred to either the Federal Ethical Committee or the South African Medical and Dental Council for further investigation (SAMJ 1983).

STRUCTURE OF PATIENTS

The Registrar of Medical Schemes (1984) has indicated the following membership statistics in respect of 228 medical aids, various benefit and 52 exempted schemes as at 31 December, 1983.

Members + Dependants (Beneficiaries)	Med Aid Schemes	Benefit Schemes	Exempt Schemes	Total
Blacks	313 703	115 130	195 057	623 890
Coloureds	316 862	74 475	263 716	655 053
Indians	145 735	6 012	82 305	234 052
Whites	2 761 096	342 658	438 092	3 541 846
Totals	3 537 396	538 275	979 170	5 054 841

ACCOUNTING PROCEDURES IN TERMS OF THE MEDICAL SCHEMES ACT

The nature of the statutory legislation governing medical aid insurance in South Africa has an impact on the accounting methods used by every private practitioner, even though he may choose to conduct his affairs outside the system by charging private fees.

Rendition of Accounts and Mandatory Documentation

The information to be specified on accounts and the manner in which they are to be rendered are prescribed by regulation in terms of the Medical Schemes Act. The procedures are quite specific and must be followed in every case where services are rendered to members of medical aid schemes, irrespective of whether statutory fees are being charged with a view to receiving direct payment from the scheme, or where the patient is to be personally responsible for settling his own account at private rates. In the latter case, the medical scheme is obliged to re-imburse the member with whatever amount it would have paid the practitioner had the services been rendered at the scale of benefit rate, but will only do so if the account is fully specified and submitted in accordance with the prescribed regulations. Even accounts for "private" medical aid patients must, therefore, conform in such manner for the sake of maintaining good relationships.

Certain medical schemes may accept direct submission of accounts by special arrangement with the practitioner. In all other cases accounts must in the first instance be rendered to the patient within 30 days of treatment and contain the following information:

* surname and initials of the member;
* the first name of the patient as specified on his membership card;
* the name of the scheme;
* the membership number of the member;
* the practice code number;
* the date on which each service was rendered;
* the nature and cost of each service;
* the procedure or service code;
* certification by way of a rubber stamp if the account is a photo-copy;
* a statement of whether the services have been charged according to the scale of benefits;
* the name of the referring practitioner in the case of specialist services.

Overdue Accounts for Direct Submission to Medical Schemes

In terms of the prescribed regulations, medical schemes are obliged to effect direct payment to a private practitioner within six weeks of receiving a valid account for.services rendered to any of their members at the scale of benefit rate.

If, however, the account remains unpaid for 90 days, the third account may be sent directly to the scheme by certified mail and clearly marked " Overdue - Please Investigate". Under these circumstances, the scheme is compelled to either settle the account or furnish sound reasons as to why it refuses to do so. The practitioner's recourse in the event of him not being satisfied in such a situation is to lodge a complaint with the Registrar of Medical Schemes who will then investigate on his behalf.

Procedure and Diagnosis Codes

Procedure codes have been established in respect of virtually every item which is charged on a fee for service basis and form an integral part of the scale of benefit tariff that is promulgated from time to time. A diagnosis must also be specified in the case of all consultations and visits. Although diagnosis codes are not prescribed by legislation, they are generally used in conjunction with computer systems and services for ease of input.

Authentication of Patients

Medical schemes issue all members with cards which include the names of any dependants as proof of membership. Practitioners can insist on patients producing their cards in order to obtain services at the scale of benefit rates, but seldom do so because of difficulties which may subsequently arise.

MEDICAL DOCUMENTATION

Apart from the Department of Health and Welfare being notified of the occurrence of specifically prescribed diseases, there are no mandatory regulations dealing with medical documentation as such.

Most practitioners maintain an efficient clinical record-keeping system for the purposes of both sound patient management and in the unlikely event of a medico-legal enquiry. There are in fact very few lawsuits against the medical profession in South Africa.

STATUTORY BODIES

Certain functions in respect of health matters have been entrusted to statutory bodies whose constitutions, powers and functions are laid down by various Acts of Parliament. Some of these are described below.

The South African Medical and Dental Council (SAMDC) was constituted in 1928 and its main functions can be summarised as follows:

* control the training, practice, and standards of conduct of medical practitioners, dentists, the supplementary health services professions and to assist in promoting the health of the population at large; all such practitioners are compelled to register with the Council;

* establish and maintain registers in respect of the specialities of medical practitioners and dentists under conditions prescribed by the Minister of Health and Welfare on its recommendation;

* investigate complaints with regard to misdemeanours or excessive fees for services rendered by registered persons and take disciplinary measures where indicated;

* submit recommendations to the Minister relating to the minimum curricula at training institutions and the degrees required to obtain registration with the Council.

The Central Council for Medical Schemes was established to:

* control, promote and co-ordinate the establishment, development and functioning of medical schemes;
* investigate and settle disputes arising from the activities of registered medical schemes;
* submit recommendations to the Minister of Health prescribing the requirements with which medical schemes must comply from time to time.

Other statutory bodies include:

* The Representative Association of Medical Schemes which, inter alia, is responsible for determining the statutory scale of benefits in conjunction with the Medical Association as prescribed for by the Medical Schemes Act.
* The Medical Research Council whose policy is to support medical research at various institutions, universities and hospitals.
* The South African Institute for Medical Research which includes diagnostic laboratory services, production and teaching amongst its various functions.
* The South African Pharmacy Board.
* The South African Nursing Council.
* The South African Nursing Association.
* The Dental Mechanicians Board.
* The Medicines Control Council.
* The National Air Pollution Advisory Committee.

PROFESSIONAL ORGANISATIONS

The following is but a brief list of the innumerable societies and associations connected with medicine and health care.

* The Medical Association of South Africa which is the official spokesman for doctors in the country. Membership is voluntary but restricted to persons registered with the South African Medical and Dental Council.
* The College of Medicine of South Africa.
* The National General Practitioners Group of MASA.
* The Pharmaceutical Society of South Africa.
* The South African Academy of Family Practice / Primary Care.
* The South African Medical Informatics Group.
* The South African Society of Physiotherapy.

COMPUTER SUPPORT

Bearing in mind that focus is being concentrated on private general practice, the benefits of using computers in this area are universal and well-known. The types of systems supported in South Africa are no doubt similar to those in other countries which have medical aid insurance structured on a direct payment plan or a re-imbursive basis.

Perhaps the stringent requirements of the Medical Schemes Act are unique and that this is a contributory factor to the relatively high usage of computers by general practitioners in the country.

Systems Available

The systems are almost exclusively confined to practice administration and can be divided between the two main categories of bureau services that have been in existence since the early 1970's, and the more recent in-house microcomputers.

There are isolated instances of remote data-entry systems linked via modem to central mainframes, but real time on-line technology as such is not available to general practitioners.

The main application areas are patient accounting and financial control systems. There is an increasing use of other packages, however, such as word processing, appointment scheduling and dispensary stock control.

Attempts have been made to implement clinical record-keeping systems with little success.

Penetration

Although there are no accurate statistics available, it is generally accepted that approximately 27 to 32 percent of private general practitioners in South Africa are making use of computer technology and that this is more or less evenly distributed between bureau services and microcomputers.

There are less than 10 service bureaux and upwards of 50 microcomputer vendors in operation. Of the innumerable microcomputer patient accounting packages that have been in and out of the market since its inception, there are about a dozen which have now matured and gained general acceptance.

Problems

The problems experienced in South Africa after the arrival of microcomputers have certainly not been confined to the unreliable hardware and ineffective software which were mostly prevalent in the earlier days.

An understandable difficulty stems from the doctor's general lack of expertise in the area of business management. This is now compounded by insufficient knowledge relating to computer technology in many cases, and how to evaluate the advantages or disadvantages of the different microcomputer packages and bureau services that are available. All too often systems are acquired without any feasibility having been carried and then price becomes the main deciding factor.

On the other hand, a bandwagon situation has developed with the usual number of unqualified and unscrupulous vendors exploiting the market. The South African computer industry is devoid of any formal system of accreditation. Although the Business Equipment Association has established a Computer Dealers Division with its own code of ethics, membership is voluntary and few suppliers of medical systems are members.

Successful installations during the first two years of microcomputers were few and far between. The disaster stories are diminishing, but there are still a number of over-ambitious claims being made by over-zealous vendors which not only creates market confusion, but also leads to a high incidence of dissatisfied users.

Software piracy is also a source of concern and recommendations for the introduction of satisfactory legislation will soon be presented to government by representative organisations of the computer industry.

Data Transmission

As at 31 March there were 48 377 data modems in service. All three of the recognised methods of data transmission are used, i.e. dial-up operation via the public switched telephone network, leased line working, and the use of a public switched data network, known as SAPONET. This network has been in use since April 1979, providing circuit switching service at user speeds up to and including 9600 bits per second.

During February, 1982, SAPONET was equipped to provide packet-switching service in addition to circuit switching. The network access protocol used is in accordance with the 1980 version of CCITT recommendation X.25, providing packet-switching service at user speeds of up to and including 64000 bits per second. The network has also been equipped with overseas packet-switching links and international packet-switching is available to countries like the United States of America, the United Kingdom, Belgium, France, Japan, Spain, Switzerland, West Germany and Australia.

The Triple-X PAD service, which allows asynchronous users access to the packet-switching services, is available. The packet-switching service was extended to country areas during 1984/85 (South African Foundation 1986).

TRENDS AND FUTURE DEVELOPMENTS

Local research into the comparative performance of stand-alone micros versus conventional bureau services in different types of practices, the development of local area networks, the feasibility of on-line communication to central mainframes providing information data-banks, the impact of BELTEL, the future potential for computers in private practice - particularly with regard to clinical applications - indicate:

* the need for information to run a successful practice is greater now than ever before; computerisation in one form or another is largely restricted to patient accounting at present, but applications such as general ledger, financial modelling and word processing are gaining acceptance;

* the question of switching from a bureau to an in-house micro should be evaluated from time to time as circumstances indicate;

* establishing sound decision criteria based on present and future needs is vital for the success of changing from one system or supplier to another;

* there is only limited use of on-line communication systems by private practices at present, but this is expected to grow within the next two years;

* medical information databases are being developed in South Africa, but how and when they will be made available has yet to be announced;

* bureaux will have to expand their range of services and assist in preparing clients for the increased use of on-line technology that is expected during the next two to five years;

* clinical applications represent a most exciting area for development, but it is unlikely that they will be widely used in private practice for some years to come;

* although computer awareness is increasing among members of the medical profession, a clear understanding of the computer's full potential and the implications of alternative methodologies, is generally lacking;

* Herbst (1984) concludes that those who view the computer only as a storage and retrieval device, or merely as an administrative tool, are losing out on its full potential to improve qualitative aspects of medical care.

Digressing from private practice in conclusion, research and development is taking place in the area of expert systems for primary and ambulatory care specifically for Third World conditions. Amongst these is a computerised diagnostic program for primary health care, "SASEP", which was described at the South African Medical Informatics Congress (Briggs et al 1984). Hanmer (1984) has also reviewed the overall implications of medical informatics for developing countries.

Apart from the fact that the computer industry itself is so dynamic, there are many forces at work both inside and outside South Africa which would have a profound effect on all aspects of the country's future. These include far-reaching constitutional changes at government level, the economy, threatened embargoes and many more.

Results arising out of current investigations into the privatisation of health care may lead to the establishment of Health Maintenance Organisations at a later date, and this would naturally bring about major changes to the entire structure described in this paper.

REFERENCES

Benatar SR, Saven AM (1985).Morbidity Trends in the Medical Wards at Groote Schuur Hospital - 1971 and 1982. SA Med J 15 June, 1985.

Briggs BR, Javett SL, Pistorious GJ, van den Berg ADP, de Klerk JN (1984) SASEP, A Computerised Diagnostic Program for Primary Health Care. Paper presented at SAMIG Congress, Cape Town 1985.

Bureau of Financial Analysis (1984). The Structure and Income/Cost Structure of the General Practitioner in the Republic of South Africa, University of Pretoria 1984.

Department of Health and Welfare. Report of the Director-General for Health and Welfare for the Year 1984.

Guide to The Health Act, Act No. 63, 1977. Pretoria 1978.

Hanmer LA, (1985). Medical Informatics for Developing Countries. Paper presented at SAMIG Congress, Cape Town 1985.

Herbst AJ (1985). How Medical Doctors in South Africa Perceive Computers. Paper presented at SAMIG Congress, Cape Town 1985

Nel PD (1984). Community Involvement in Health Care. SA Cont Med Educ J, Vol 2 No 4. April 1984.

Registrar of Medical Schemes Annual Report, 1984. Annexures 1 and 2.

Retief FP (1984). Address at the Fourth Interdisciplinary Symposium of The College of Medicine, Durban 1984.

SAMJ (1983). News from the Secretariat, Cost Awareness/Peer Review. SA Med J, 12 November 1983.

Smith JA (1981). The Day Hospitals Organisation. SA Med J, April 1981.

South Africa Foundation, 1986 Information Digest.

South Africa 1985. Official Yearbook of the Republic of South Africa, 1985. Eleventh Edition - 1985, Department of Foreign Affairs 1985.

Spencer IWF (1984). Primary Care in South Africa, SA Cont Med Educ J, Vol 2 No 4. April 1984.

THE HEALTH CARE SYSTEM OF THE FEDERAL REPUBLIC OF GERMANY

J.R. Möhr

Institut für Medizinische Dokumentation, Statistik und Datenverarbeitung der Universität Heidelberg
Im Neuenheimer Feld 325, D-6900 Heidelberg

History

In every country probably, the health care system and other social systems are less an effect of a response to objective needs than of historic development. The historic development of the F.R.G. was profoundly determined by her central location in Europe. It shaped the structure and functioning of the society that we find there today. While in the North there is a fecund and flat country which supports large estates, the South is characterized by hilly and mountainous sites where people had to toil hard for their lives. In addition, all areas were again and again swept by successions of tribes of different origins in the past.

The ethnic differences and differences of the environment produced substantial regional differences in the economy, laws and habits. Therefore the Federal Republic of Germany has to account in many ways for the requirements of the different regional systems of the eleven constituent states. And this, of course, reflects in the health care system. The fact that we have a democratic but also a particularistic and liberalistic society affects the health care system, the educational system and the legislation more than private industry, science and research.

This has the consequence that many of the important subsystems of the health care system and many of the subsystems affecting it are all diversified regionally, socially or otherwise. This influences the organization of physicians, sick funds, hospital providers as well as universities, employers, unions and, of course, communities.

The health care system was decisively shaped around a hundred years ago, when a German nation had been united in the form of an Empire under the King of Prussia and the Chancellor Bismarck.

Around 1820 already, the Prussians had first instituted some laws limiting the work hours for children. The reason was at that time that the demand of the army for young and healthy men could not be met because in some areas the country's youth was literally spoiled by work days lasting up to 16 hours. So there was some tradition with respect to social legislation when Bismarck proposed to his Emperor in the late 1870ies what later became the Impirial Insurance Act (Reichsversicherungsordnung). The dominating motive this time seems to have been the attempt to limit the attractiveness of the socialist movement under the leadership of people like Marx and Engels.

The Insurance System

The legislation begun with the insurance act of 1883, was finalized around the turn of the century and eventually required all persons below a certain income limit to be insured against accidents, disease and disability (compulsory insurance). This insurance was based on the solidarity principle in contrast to most of the private insurances existing already at that time. The solidarity principle signifies that the contribution of an insured person is related to its means rather than to the risk of the insured good. The latter is the case in the private insurance which is based upon the equivalence principle. Also in the compulsory insurance, 50 % of the premiums are paid by the employer.

Another characteristic of this insurance system is that a multiplicity of sick funds is made available. Some of them had been in existence already in 1883, others were newly installed since. In this way regional and social differences could be accounted for. These sick funds had a considerable administrative autonomy from the beginning on.

The number of sick funds is substantial with a total of over 1,300. There are close to 300 community defined local sick funds. Almost 900 are made available by companies to their employees, 150 by trade guilds. A few sick funds are available for workers and for employees as subsidy to the compulsory sick funds. These are relatively important since they have a large number of members.

Approximately 50 % of the insured population are members of local sick funds. More than a quarter - mostly waged employees - are members of subsidiary sick funds. Less than a quarter are distributed over the remaining sick funds, in particular the large number of company sick funds.

These sick funds generally have a two level administration consisting of an assembly of deputies and a board of directors which are composed equally of representatives of employers and employees. This administration is supported by a staff of executives. The duty of this administration is to decide the fund's policy, the kind and quality of services offered and to negotiate fees with the various providers of medical care services.

Much of this is, of course, to be decided with the narrow limits of federal and state laws and with basic directions of policies established by the associations of various types of sick funds.

In this way, the system of 'partitioned health insurance' of the F.R.G. is supposed to provide an attractive variation of different alternatives and to ensure optimal representation of the requirements of varying sectors of the insured population.

Relevant Organization of Private Physicians

On the other hand, this system of particularistic health insurance did have a decisive influence on many other aspects of other components of the health care system. For instance, initially the doctors would sign agreements with individual sick funds to treat their patients according to defined fees while treating the so-called 'private patients' on an honorary basis adjusting their fees to the means of the patient.

As a greater and greater percentage of the population became covered by the sick funds, the treatment of the insured patients became the dominant source of income for physicians, and negotiations with sick funds became a crucial task.

In this situation the physicians formed associations, associations of sick fund related physicians or 'Kassenärztliche Vereinigung (K.V.)'.
These K.V.s were again organized regionally and have their autonomous administration.

In the twenties these associations were finally granted the monopoly for curative care of ambulatory patients. This monopoly comprised the responsibility for establishing adequate care facilities - i.e. insuring an adequate density of physicians' practices and the right to negotiate fees for physicians' services.

Relation of Ambulatory Care and Inpatient Care

One important side effect of the monopoly of the K.V.s for curative care was in our country that the care processes for inpatients and outpatients became institutionally separated. Today a patient needing hospital care is transferred from the care of a physician or surgeon working in a private practice into the responsibility of a different team of physicians being employed by and therefore operating on the basis of a hospital. 'Attending physicians' (Belegärzte) who out of a private practice care for their patients while these are in a hospital are a possible but rather uncommon occurrence in this country. The separation of hospital care and ambulatory care entails, of course, a considerable communication between doctors in hospitals and private practices and this in turn is one of the primary concerns of health information science in our country.

Patients may sign up with one or several physicians of their choice for ambulatory care, although continuous care through family physicians and transferral to specialists through them are advocated. Family physicians are mostly practitioners (physicians not specialized in general medicine), physicians for general medicine, and to some extent also internists and pediatricians.

Transferral to a hospital has to be recommended through a practicing physician (generalist or specialist). Thus the secondary care sector is composed of hospitals and specialists.
Transferral may be directed immediately to a tertiary care institution, e.g. a university hospital.

Physician Density

Until the sixties, the K.V.s had the power to limit the number of practices in a given region. This had, of course, the effect of ensuring excellent possibilities of income for the members of the K.V.s. In the early sixties, a federal court judgement ruled that every physician who fulfilled the necessary medical qualification, had the right to open up a practice wherever he or she felt this to be suitable. This lead to a gradual but steady increase of physician density (see Fig. 2).

Currently, the number of physicians in this country exceeds 170,000 (see Fig. 2). Less than 80 % of them are active in patient care, the others in research, industry, administration, etc. if they did not cease to work or are currently unemployed. Of those involved in patient care, less than 50 % work in private practice. In this respect a substantial change has occurred over the past 50 years. In the thirties approximately 80 % of some 40,000 physicians worked out of private practice. Their total number of close to 40,000 has barely doubled since (Fig. 1). The number of physicians working in hospitals, on the other hand, has increased from a few thousand to close to 80,000. Those working in private practice can be divided almost evenly among general practitioners (specialists for family medicine) and specialists. Among the latter, internists, gynecologists, pediatricians and surgeons form the largest groups. Other specialists are ophthalmologists, oto-rhino-laryngologists, orthopedists, radiologists, etc.. Dental care requires also a medical specialization. It is, however, from the basic training of students on completely separated from other disciplines of human health care.

Fig. 1:

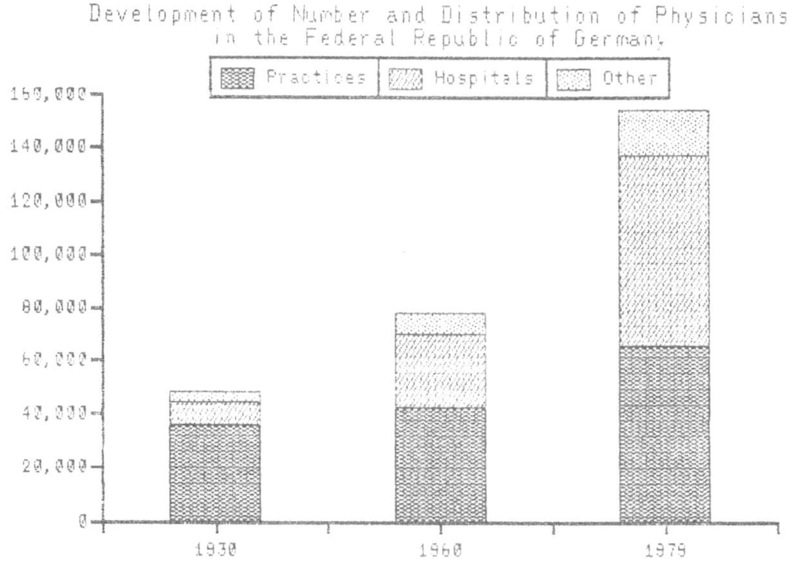

Due to the excellent social standing of the medical profession and the expectations of income, the attractiveness of the medical education is great. Currently we are forced - frequently again by court rule - to admit more than 12,000 medical students annually. The number of approbations - the approbation giving the physician the right to practice self responsibly - has attained the number of 9,000 per year. On the other hand, the number of physicians giving up active care lies in the range of 3 - 4,000 annually only. So we are heading towards a physician density which will probably outpass that of any other country in the world (Fig. 2).
It is a matter of debate whether we can put so many physicians reasonably to work.

In the past, there has been a significant shift from a predominance of physicians in private practice to a predominance of physicians employed in hospitals and other dependent positions. The latter

Fig. 2:

Trends in Physician Density

Period	Additions	Reductions	Net Increase
1976 - 81	16,200	10,400	5,800
1981 - 86	18,500	9,700	8,800
1986 - 91	19,300	8,000	11,300

fraction currently exceeds the former while in the thirties only some 20 % of physicians were salaried employees. Also the number of physicians not active in patient care has increased considerably. These colleagues work in industry, administration, scientific institutions and the like (see Fig. 1).

The increase of physicians in hospitals is due to an increased demand for hospital care as an effect of the development of morbidity as well as medical means.

Another factor affecting the need for physicians is legislation reducing over time work for physicians in hospitals. At present, it has mainly been achieved that over time work is paid for. However, legislation is expected to limit the amount of overtime. So it could be that in effect we will be glad in a couple of years to have a sufficient number of physicians available to compensate for the reduction of work hours of individual physicians.

Physicians' Earnings

I doubt, however, that it will be possible to maintain the current levels of income for physicians.

Currently, the earnings of a physician in private practice lie in a range which - depending on the specialty - is on the average 30 to 300 % above that of physicians employed in hospitals (Fig. 3). Another illustration of the level of income of physicians in private practice may be given by mentioning that the income of physicians in free practice is approximately 9 levels of income above that of employed physicians if one takes as comparison the levels of income customary for civil servants in leading positions.

Chiefs of staff employed in secondary or tertiary care hospitals may be granted permission to participate in the curative care for the patients of sick funds as if acting in private practice. Thereby they generate at times substantial income in addition to their salaries.

Over the past years, the income of physicians had a disparate development. That of general practitioners and pediatricians stayed pretty much at the same level with a slight tendency towards decrease. These specialties account for 60 - 70 % of all physicians. High technology oriented specialties like radiology and nuclear medicine still exhibit a steady increase in income even in recent years.

Fig. 3:

Physician's Earnings

(Adjusted Figures)

	Gross Returns TDM	Cost %	Gross Earnings TDM
Practice Based Physicians			
General Medicine	240	42.7	144
Internists	335	46	181
Pediatricians	203	43	116
Radiologists	619	57	269
all groups	273	43	156
Employed Physicians ('A 16')			85
Civil Servants (Leading Position)			
('B1') Director & Professor			87
('B9') Ministerial Director			163

Ambulatory Care Reimbursement System

The reimbursement system (Fig. 4) in ambulatory care is rather complicated. It involves four parties:

- patients (insured persons),
- physicians,
- the associations of sick fund related physicians, and
- sick funds.

Between these groups and institutions two inverse streams of

- securities, and
- services and remuneration

interact.

The insured members have a contract with their insurance company which entitles them to receive medical care.

The sick funds distribute claim checks among their members. If these require services from physicians they pass their claim check on to them. The physician treats the patient and notes all services and related diagnoses rendered on the claim check. The claim check also contains some identification data of the patient and the insured person - usually the earning member of the family. Four times per year, all claim checks are sorted in every practice and passed on to the K.V.. The K.V. captures the data and passes the claim checks on to the diverse sick funds.

Fig. 4: **Ambulatory Care Reimbursement System in F.R.G.**

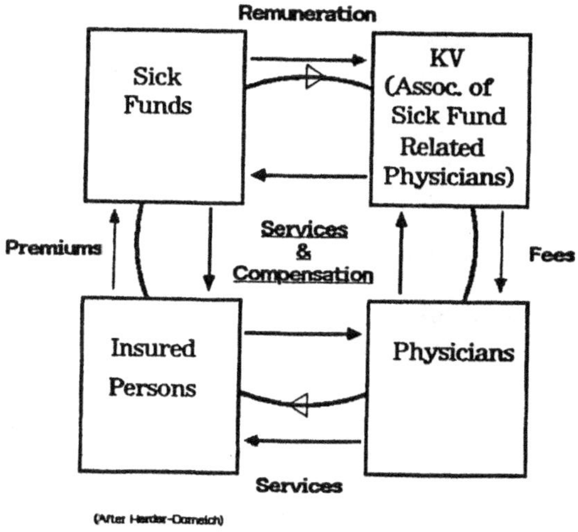

Inversely the sick funds transfer the money for the services rendered for their clients on the basis of the service documented on the claim checks to the K.V.. The K.V. distributes the money among the physicians who rendered the services. The sick funds of course generate the money through premiums from their members and the members' employers.

Significance of the Reimbursement System

The system may seem complicated. But it is necessary because it eases the task of the individual physician for whom it would be quite a burden to deal with potentially over a thousand sick funds on an individual basis.

On the one hand, the system is crucial for the K.V. in order to fulfill its duty of providing adequate and economic medical care to the population. Evaluation of the claim checks is an important means for controlling health care economy. Physicians constantly face the possibility of their return being cut down through the K.V. if they generate a quantitatively or qualitatively untypical spectrum of services.

On the other hand, the system also tends to obscure the situation. It takes usually several months before a physician is informed of the income he generated. Also the sick funds have a hard time in controlling what they spent their money for. Their situation is particularly complicated since the sick funds not only have to deal with a number of K.V.s but also with an even greater number of providers of hospital care, with pharmacies and many other institutions providing medical supplies, such as opticians, suppliers of prosthetic devices and so on.

Public Health Agencies

An important part of what in WHO terms is referred to as primary health care is executed by public health agencies (Gesundheitsämter) in the F.R.G.. These are organized either as institutions of the communities or of the states and are responsible for

- registering defined communicable diseases
- supervising hygienic standards in public facilities such as
  - kitchens and restaurants
  - water supply facilities
  - waste dumps etc.
- screening of populations, e.g.
  - radiographic screening
  - screening of school children
- execution of preventive measures, e.g.
  - vaccinations
  - maternity and child care
- determination of disability status in questionable cases (e.g. of absenteeism).

The responsibility of the health care agencies does specifically not include responsibility for curative medicine. There exist over 380 such public health agencies, employing close to 18.000 staff including 4.000 doctors.

Occupational Medicine

Another important pillar of primary health care are institutions of occupational medicine. During the last part of the 19th century, a number of large industrial companies began to offer some kind of health care to their workers and employees as part of their social services. But only in 1974 did such services become mandatory for companies of a certain size (the current interpretation being companies employing 100 persons).

These occupational health care services may be organized in one of three ways:

- through contracts with private physicians with a specialization in occupational medicine (in addition to any other specialty)
- through contract with an occupational health care center run by a professional association ('Berufsgenossenschaft', an association of employers of a defined industry, e.g. chemical industry, insuring employees and workers against work related disabilities and accidents)
- through establishment of occupational health care centers of their own.

The responsibilities comprise among others:

- diagnostic investigations concerning work abilities
- periodic screening for adverse effects
- monitoring occupational hygienic conditions in the various work environments, and making related recommendations
- recording and evaluating health care data.

As in the case of the health care agencies, the responsibility for cure is specifically exempt from the duties of occupational health care centers, due to the monopoly of the K.V.s for curative care. However, occupational health care centers are equipped for a certain amount of first aid care, which may include minor surgery.

Emergency Room Services

A final component in primary medical care are emergency room services provided by secondary and tertiary care hospitals, especially during the off duty hours of practicing physicians. Approaches in computer systems regarding these facilities are governed by the information systems in tertiary care environments and will not be covered in this article.

Hospital Care

There are over 3.000 hospitals available in our country and approximately three quarters of a million hospital beds, most of them for acute care patients. These hospitals are almost evenly divided among public, charitable and private institutions as providers of hospital care. However, hospitals provided by the public sector - usually the communities or the states - tend to be larger than private hospitals.

During the last 10 years, the number of patients treated in hospitals increases by some 20 % and the average length of stay decreased by the same percentage. Since the first days in a hospital are particularly labour intensive, this shift means an increase in the work load and generated costs. Together with a tendency to limit the amount of over time work for health care personnel, this means a considerable increase in the staff of hospitals. This development will probably continue.

Nursing Profession

In our country there are comparatively few nurses and orderlies involved in patient care - at least relative to the population. Most of this patient care personnel is active in hospitals. Their number has increased tremendously during this century. But even greater was the qualitative change with respect to the concept of nursing care as a profession. At the beginning of this century nurses were mostly part of religious or charitable organizations. They were available almost 24 hours a day for little more than the mercy of god. Today nurses are much more professionally oriented. Highly specialized skills are demanded from them and their right to regular working hours is no longer questioned.

Primary health care also relies to some extent on nurses employed by communities. The benefits of their services are enjoyed by many elderly, disabled and helpless people. The services are not very expensive and hence little remarked by the public or academia (including the author).

A big difference to nursing in some other countries is, that the nursing profession is considered a strictly non academic profession, based on a three year education with predominantly practical orientation and approximately 1.500 hours of theoretical instruction. We do not have academically qualified nurses.

Hospital Cost

The nursing staff and the medical staff account for much of the personnel costs in a hospital, which make up close to 70 % of hospital costs, while drugs and other medical supplies account for approximately half of the remaining costs only (Fig. 5).

Fig. 5:

Sick Fund Expenditures 1983

Inpatient Care	32 %
Ambulatory Care	18 %
Drugs	15 %
Dental Care	7 %
Dental Prosthetics	7 %
Cash	6 %
Remedial Devices	5 %
Maternal Care	3 %
Death Subsidy	2 %
Administration	4 %
Total Expenditures	95.7 Billion DM

The total cost lies in the range of 250 DM per day of patient care, including doctor's fees and medical care. In maximal care facilities like university hospitals it amounts to around as to DM 400 (in 1984).

Reimbursement of Hospitals

So far the remuneration of hospitals has been based on a flat rate per day of patient care. This rate determined by dividing the costs of the hospital by the number of care days rendered. The result is subject to negotiations between the federations of the sick funds and the providers of hospital care or even individual hospitals.

This regimen in itself is by some presumed to account for the comparatively long time that our patients stay in the hospital. Most costs are generated in the initial phase of a hospital stay through intensive diagnosis and treatment. Towards the end of a hospitalization period the costs generated through treatment tend to be considerably below average. Therefore, if a patient is kept a couple of days longer his kind of treatment actually represents a gain over that of a new patient who could replace him. Because the patient in this stage generates fewer costs than a new patient and even less than the returns are per patient day, he actually generates income for the hospital in this phase.

In this respect, however, new developments are under way. Since January 1st, 1986, hospitals have to convert to prospective budget orientation. It also is likely that in the future the reimbursement system will differentiate between different categories of morbidity, probably similar to the 'Diagnosis Related Grouping' of patients adopted in the United States of America.

Drug Situation

The number of drugs that we can choose from in the F.R.G. is high. The items contained in some of the more renowned drug data bases range between 14.000 and 140.000. Estimates of pharmacists that I have consultated point in the direction of 30.000 drugs that are available if one includes homeopathic drugs and nature cure remedies.

The total spectrum of drugs used by a given physician per quarter lies in the range of 3.000. The number kept in a typical hospital pharmacy is in the range of 1.500. The 95% spectrum of the most frequently used drugs in a general physician's office is in the range of 6 to 800 different specialties. Just to complete this sequence I might add that some physicians in the Netherlands claim to be able to treat effectively with only 60 to 80 different specialties.

The large number of drugs available in the F.R.G. is provided by roughly 1.000 producers and distributed predominantly through close to 15.000 pharmacies. The annual expenditures of over 9 billion DM amount to some 15 % of sick fund expenditures.

Sick fund expenditures totaled close to 100 billion DM in 1984. 50% of this were spent on hospitals' and physicians' bills (32 and 18 % respectively). Hospital care expenditures were nearly twice as high as ambulatory care expenditures. Drugs account for the third largest sector in expenses, or for some 15 %. As in other countries, these costs have been rising over the past years, so that they amount to more than 10 % of the GNP.

Status of Computer Support

Computer support in health care has attained a notable extent in the F.R.G. so far. The developments focus clearly on the support of hospitals and to a lesser extent on that of practicing physicians. The employment of computers in public health agencies is limited to a few instances of involvement in the support and maintenance of health registries and to some simple isolated applications like text processing. Industrial health care centers do to a much greater extent profit from computer support, in several instances based on the extensive computer facilities of the companies running the health care center.

Almost all hospitals do employ computers to some extent, predominantly for the support of administrative functions. In several instances fairly sophisticated and comprehensive integrated computer systems have evolved over the years. These may include support of emergency room services but are usually not available to private physicians.

With respect to the private physicians a rather peculiar situation exists. The great market potential attracts more and more companies. The situation is characterized by enormous dynamics. Currently (1986) there are probably more than 150 systems available on the market (Fig. 6). These share probably less than 2.000 installations. Only some 1.500 practices have been registered as using computers for the processing of their claim checks - the most frequent application and one requiring official acceptance through the K.V..

Therefore the penetration has reached mere 2 % of the total of 70.000 practices. Three vendors share 40 % of this market.

It seems not unlikely to me that the early endeavours in this field in our country which involved frequently rather immature systems as well as endeavours from various interest groups to control and direct these developments are not unrelated to this comparative failure to succeed so far.

Fig. 6:

STATUS OF COMPUTER SUPPORT

~ 130 VENDORS OF RVO COMPATIBLE BILLING AND DOCUMENTATION SYSTEMS

~ 3 VENDORS SHARING 40 % OF MARKET
- SUPERVISION THROUGH "CENTRAL INSTITUTE OF KBV" -

~ 1100 OFFICES REGISTERED (1-2 % OF 70.000)

~ 20 % INCREASE SINCE 1984

The functions of these systems focus on the support of administrative procedures:

- patient registration
- capture of services and diagnoses
- claim check processing and billing
- support of some fundamental statistics.

More sophisticated systems tend to feature functions such as:

- support of medical documentation
- automated generation of reports and prescriptions
- data bases and query facilities
- automated checking, reminders etc..

In comparison with systems from other countries the virtual absence of decision support features in the form of knowledge bases and similar AI approaches, the lack of sophistication with respect to the support of scientific evaluations and the lack of statistical analysis systems is conspicuous.

Costs of the systems have decreased in recent years. 'Introductory versions' of systems are currently offered in the 20 - 30.000 DM range. Reliable professional configurations are still likely to cost at least twice as much. These figures apply to office based in-house systems. Large shared facilities have never been developed to any significant extent and are currently not used in this country in private practice.

Current Issues in Health Care

Logically, attempts to curb the cost development in health care constitute a focus of attention. Proposed measures include substituting ambulatory care for hospital care, reducing the consumption of drugs as well as altering the reimbursement procedures. Much concern is also meeting the growing number of physicians since some investigations suggest that any number of physicians is able to survive and generate at least a moderate income.

Other current concerns of health care policy are, of course, the improvement of health services. Several research programmes have been established in order to improve technical services, to learn more about the health care systems and to find means for modifying it.

An interesting institution has been installed in 1978 and became part of our health care related legislature in order to assist in the direction of health care policy. It is the 'concerted action in health care' or 'Konzertierte Aktion im Gesundheitswesen'.

Under the direction of the Federal Ministry for Work and Social Affairs representatives of all institutions involved in health care convene twice yearly in order to discuss health policy issues. The list of represented bodies is quite long and comprehensive and includes physicians' organizations, sick funds, communities, employers and trade unions. The goals are to elaborate proposals for determining the goals of health care - economically and medically - and to work out suggestions for rationalization and improvement. The concerted action has no executive powers. Its value is debated. It seems to me to be a worthwhile concept and institution.

With this I would like to conclude this overview of the German health care system. It would have been appropriate to begin this type of a presentation with a list of disclaimers. Of course it is impossible to touch all aspects of a complex system such as the health care system of a nation. All one should expect from a presentation of this kind is to serve as a piece of reference - an impressionistic picture which might perhaps highlight by contrast some aspects of the personal experience of some readers, that of some others by similarity. In this respect I hope to have met the expectations.

Selected References

Anonym: Jahrbuch 78/79 (Hartmannbund, Verband der Ärzte Deutschlands, 1979).

Arnold, M., Brauer, H.P., Deneke, J.F.V., Fiedler, E.: Der Beruf des Arztes in der Bundesrepublik Deutschland. (Köln, Deutscher Ärzteverlag: 1984).

Bundesminister für Jugend, Familie und Gesundheit: Daten des Gesundheitswesens - Ausgabe 1983 (Düsseldorf, Kohlhammer: 1983).

Hoffmann, H.: Zur Situation des Krankenhauswesens in der Bundesrepublik Deutschland. (Düsseldorf, Kohlhammer: 1985).

Möhr, J.R., Haehn, K.D.: Verdenstudie: Strukturanalyse Allgemeinmedizinischer Praxen. (Köln, Deutscher Ärzteverlag: 1977).

Möhr, J.R., Köhler, C.O. (eds.): Betriebsärztliche Informationssysteme. (Berlin, Heidelberg, New York, Springer: 1980).

Lordieck, W., Reichertz, P.L.: Die EDV in den Krankenhäusern der Bundesrepublik Deutschland. (Berlin, Heidelberg, New York, Tokyo, Springer: 1983).

Schicke, R.K.: Arzt und Gesundheitsversorgung im gesellschaftlichen Sicherungssystem. Bundesrepublik Deutschland - England - USA. (Freiburg, Rombach: 1971).

Schippgeres, H.: Entwicklung moderner Medizin. Probleme, Prognosen, Tendenzen. Schriftenreihe der Bezirksärztekammer Nordwürttemberg Nr. 10 (Stuttgart, Gentner: 1968).

Strobawa, F.F.: Die ärztlichen Organisationen in der Bundesrepublik Deutschland. (Droste: 1979).

Van Eimeren, W.: Multimorbidität in der Allgemeinpraxis. (Köln, Deutscher Ärzteverlag: 1976).

SYSTEMS ANALYSIS FOR COMPUTERS IN AMBULATORY HEALTH CARE IN IRELAND

Rory R. O'Moore,
St. James's Hospital,
Dublin 8,
Ireland,

INTRODUCTION

The Administration of the Health Services at a local level in Ireland is largely by the eight Health Boards which were established by the Health Act of 1970. The geographic distribution of these and the populations served are shown in Figure 1. The total population in 1982 was 3,483,000. (1)

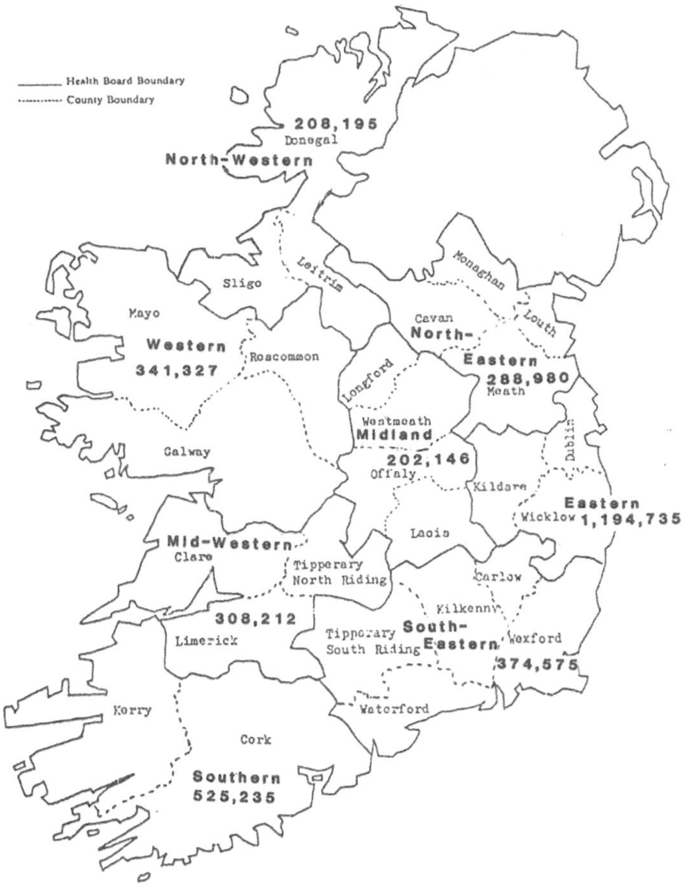

FIG.1 THE EIGHT HEALTH BOARD AREAS

Primary Health Care is delivered predominantly by doctors working within the General Medical Services (GMS). This service commenced in 1972 and replaced the previous District Medical Officers Service (**Dispensary** Doctors). Eighty per cent (80%) of the General Practitioners are involved in this scheme. The aim of which is to provide a service, for those eligible for free medical care, which would give "the greatest practical choice of doctor, and the least practicable distinction between private patients and those availing of the service".(2) This service caters for almost 40% of patients in Primary Health Care. The remaining 60% of patients are regarded as non eligible and use private primary care. The vast majority of doctors in the GMS scheme are also in private practice. In addition approximately 366 doctors are in private practice alone. (3)

TABLE 1 **General practitioner population**

Total general practitioner population	1,821
GP population (GMS)	1,455 (79·9 per cent)
GP population (private alone)	366 (20·1 per cent)

1. STRUCTURE OF PRIMARY CARE

1.1 SUPPLY

General Practitioners provide the major component of Primary Care in Ireland. In 1984 there were 1,821 General Practitioners. The doctor patient ratio is 1:1,890 with a mean GMS panel size of 888.(2) The distribution of these doctors in the different Health Boards is shown in Figure 2.

There are also some 230 doctors employed in the Community Health Services, many of whom are involved in some aspects of primary care, for example pre school and school medical examinations, immunization programmes and other aspects of preventative medicine. (4) Some 1,800 Public Health Service Nurses are also employed in the various aspects of Community Health Care. It is estimated that between 200 - 250 doctors hold part time or sessional appointments in Occupational Medicine. About 120 doctors devote at least 25% of their time to occupational medicine while about 12% of these doctors work in the specialty on a whole time basis.

The Hospital Services contribute to ambulatory care through their 'walk in' Accident and Emergency and Outpatient services. Currently there are 1,800 Junior Hospital Doctors (in training posts). A large majority of consultant staff in Hospitals are involved in ambulatory care via their outpatient clinics. The numbers of consultants concerned are:- 100 Obstetricians/ Gynaecologists, 51 Paediatricians, 184 Physicians, 201 Psychiatrists, 151 General Surgeons, 42 Orthopaedic Surgeons, 37 Ophthalmic Surgeons and 30 Ear, Nose and Throat Surgeons.(5).

FIG. 2 the general practitioner populations in their respective health board regions

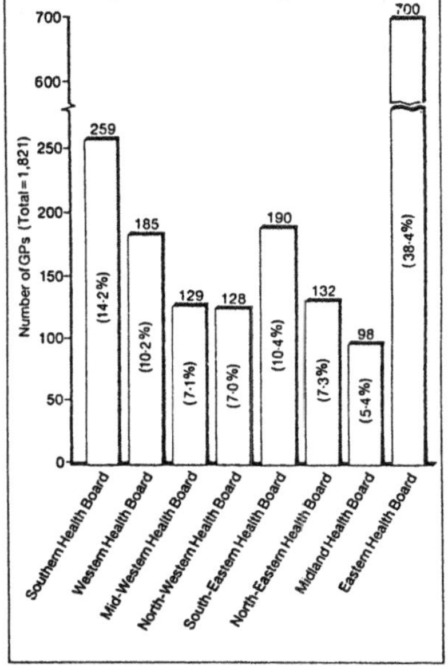

In Ireland direct consultant involvement in primary care is unusual, although some private patients may make direct contact with a consultant of choice.

The percentage of primary care spent in ambulatory care is difficult to assess. However, an estimate may be made from the GMS returns which give statistics on primary care for almost 40 per cent of the population. There were almost 8 million patient doctor contacts in 1984. Of these 1.5 million were domicillary visits. It is probably safe to assume that the pattern in the private sector (60 per cent) will be fairly comparable.

1.2 EXPENDITURE

The latest available figures on Health Expenditure are from 1983. Estimates for Capital expenditure amounted to IR £53 million. Non Capital expenditure was IR 1,033 million pounds which represents 7.77% of the Gross National Product. Only 6.5% of **this total is raised from Health Contributions, the remainder from the exchequer. (1)**

Doctors income is difficult to determine **accurately.** In 1984 the 1,463 doctors in the G.M.S. received a total of 30.25 million pounds (IR£) for primary care of the 1,299,165 (38% population) covered by the scheme. This average of IR£ 20,000 per doctor, must also cover practice expenses, locums etc. It is impossible to estimate income derived from the two million (60%) of citizens who are ineligible for the GMS. Of these some 1,033,261 are privately insured in a scheme which partly reimbures general practitioner charges.

Hospital Consultants are paid salaries averaging £20,000 for their work in the public sector. Income from private patients who are insured averaged in 1984 just below IR £20,000 per annum. (6)

Table 2 illustrates the broad headings for non capital expenditure by the various programmes in the Health Services.

TABLE 2 ESTIMATED NON CAPITAL EXPENDITURE 1983.(1)

SERVICE	MAJOR ITEMS	COST (Million IR£)
Community Protection Programme	Immunization/Child Health	16.9
Community Health Services	Home Nursing/Dental	50.5
General Medical Services	Doctors Fees/Drugs	88.6
Community Welfare	Disabled Grants/ Voluntary Agencies	83.3
Psychiatric Services	Care/Prevention	131.1
Programme for **Handicapped**	Care/Assessment	107.6
General Hospital Programme	Regional/Voluntary/ Health Boards	558.1
General Support	Administration/ Superannuation	54.1
	TOTAL	1,090.2

2. STRUCTURE OF THE POPULATION

The population and some demographic details are shown in Table 3.

TABLE 3 **POPULATION OF EACH HEALTH BOARD AREA BY AGE AND BY SEX, 1981**

	Eastern	Midland	Mid-Western	North-Eastern	North-Western	South-Eastern	Southern	Western	Ireland
Total population:	1,194,735	202,146	308,212	288,980	208,195	374,575	525,235	341,327	3,443,405
Age groups:									
Number 0-14 years	357,581	63,554	94,896	91,871	61,968	117,578	156,516	99,765	1,043,729
Number 15-44 years	544,158	80,208	124,970	117,470	78,158	150,879	213,843	130,634	1,440,320
Number 45-64 years	191,426	36,478	54,085	49,505	37,822	65,331	93,162	62,593	590,402
Number 65-74 years	65,437	13,903	22,100	19,538	19,185	25,961	40,081	30,852	237,057
Number 75 years and over	36,133	8,003	12,161	10,596	11,062	14,826	21,633	17,483	131,897
Percentage 0-14 years	29.9	31.4	30.8	31.8	29.8	31.4	29.8	29.2	30.3
Percentage 15-44 years	45.5	39.7	40.5	40.6	37.5	40.3	40.7	38.3	41.8
Percentage 45-64 years	16.0	18.0	17.5	17.1	18.2	17.4	17.7	18.3	17.1
Percentage 65-74 years	5.5	6.9	7.2	6.8	9.2	6.9	7.6	9.0	6.9
Percentage 75 years and over	3.0	4.0	3.9	3.7	5.3	4.0	4.1	5.1	3.8
Marital status (persons aged 15 years and over)									
Number Single ...	326,217	54,006	81,511	73,878	58,217	97,176	143,093	97,850	931,948
Number Married	455,932	73,901	115,256	108,435	75,462	139,650	196,299	123,165	1,288,100
Number Widowed	55,005	10,685	16,549	14,796	12,548	20,171	29,327	20,547	179,628
Percentage Single ...	39.0	39.0	38.2	37.5	39.8	37.8	38.8	40.5	38.8
Percentage Married	54.5	53.3	54.0	55.0	51.6	54.3	53.2	51.0	53.7
Percentage Widowed	6.6	7.7	7.8	7.5	8.6	7.8	8.0	8.5	7.5
Dependency ratio ... (number of persons aged 0-14 years and aged 65 years or over as a percentage of those aged 15-64 years)	62.4	73.2	72.1	73.1	79.5	73.2	71.1	76.6	69.6

Source: Central Statistics Office.

It should be noted that a high proportion (one third) of the population is under 14 years of age. Morbidity statistics are not available for the GMS scheme. Some indication of the overall population morbidity may be estimated from the various tables in "Statistical Information relevant to the Health Services"(1) which is published annually by the Department of Health. This contains summary information on chronic disease registers, notifiable diseases, psychiatric admissions, mental and physical handicap statistics etc. An example from the Medico - Social Research Board Hospital in patient enquiry scheme is shown in Table 4.

The catchment areas vary greatly. In a survey of general practice,(3) it was found that the majority of doctors in private practice only were doctors in the younger age group working in the centres of high population in the Eastern and Southern Health Board areas (a doctor may only apply for entry to the GMS after five years working in an area). The majority of other doctors in these Health Boards had large private patient lists and small (<500) GMS lists.

TABLE 4

HOSPITAL IN-PATIENT ENQUIRY: NUMBER OF DISCHARGES AND AVERAGE DURATION OF STAY BY DIAGNOSTIC CATEGORY, 1982

Diagnosis	Number of cases	%	Average duration of stay (in days)
Accidents, poisonings and violence	51,485	13.3	7.3
Diseases of the respiratory system	42,113	10.9	11.1
Diseases of the digestive system	44,315	11.4	8.1
Diseases of the circulatory system	37,612	9.7	14.6
Symptoms and ill-defined conditions	36,076	9.3	5.9
Diseases of the genito-urinary system	33,427	8.6	7.0
Special admissions and consultations	28,812	7.4	7.2
Diseases of the nervous system and sense organs ...	21,380	5.5	8.9
Neoplasms	21,164	5.5	14.4
Diseases of the musculo-skeletal system and connective tissue	18,330	4.7	11.8
Infective and parasitic diseases	12,035	3.1	10.9
Diseases of the skin and subcutaneous tissue	10,228	2.6	7.7
Endocrine, nutritional and metabolic diseases	8,440	2.3	11.3
Congenital anomalies	7,961	2.1	9.7
Diseases of the blood and blood-forming organs ...	3,785	1.0	9.7
Miscellaneous	10,769	2.8	8.9
Total	387,932	100.2	10.2

Note: The Hospital In-Patient Enquiry does not cover all discharges from hospitals. It does not cover Maternity but does cover a high percentage of the remainder of acute discharges.
Source: Hospital In-Patient Enquiry, Medico-Social Research Board.

In the other six Health Boards an inverse relationship existed between doctors with large GMS lists (1,000 - 2,000) who had low (<10%) private patient lists and those with large private patient lists (>60%) who had small GMS lists (<500).

The 60% per cent private patients select their own doctor. Patients within the GMS register with the doctor of their choice, provided he is in the GMS and is prepared to accept them. Normally the doctor must live within seven miles and have a list of less than 2,500 patients. In difficulties the Health Board arranges entry to a doctor panel.

Treatment periods in ambulatory care are defined by episode only.

3. STRUCTURE OF PRACTICE

3.1 TYPE OF PRACTICE

In a survey of General Practice (3) it was found that 63 per cent of doctors did not share premises, 37 per cent shared premises with at least one other doctor. Seventy six per cent (76%) did not have a legal partnership with another doctor. Thus the incidence of single practices is between 63 - 76 per cent. Group practices are gradually beginning to evolve in urban areas.

The majority of doctors (42 per cent) work from adapted premises separate from their residences, thirty two per cent from home and 24 per cent from purpose built premises. Self ownership of premises occurred in 65 per cent, rented accommodation was used by 20 per cent, Health Board ownership occurred in 15 per cent of practices. These latter were often in a Health Centre also utilized by community physicians, public health nurses and social workers, usually in rural areas.

The percentages of doctors in different types of practice are illustrated in Table 5. Urban practice (>5,000 population) was the most frequent type in the Eastern (72 per cent) and Southern (45 per cent) Health Boards. Rural practices dominated the other Health Board areas with the exception of the Mid Western (37 per cent urban, 37 per cent rural) and Midland which was 53 per cent mixed.

Hospital outpatient clinics are run in almost all the larger Hospitals.

TABLE 5 **Practice areas (urban area defined as one with a population of 5,000 or more)**

	Percentage
Mainly urban	42·1
Mainly rural	31·1
Mixed	26·8
	100·0

3.2 USAGE

No figures are available for private ambulatory care but some estimate of relative usage of general practitioner versus outpatient clinic ambulatory care may be obtained by inspection of Tables 6 and 7. In this context it should be mentioned that 85% of the population are eligible for free hospital services including specialist outpatients clinics. From these figures it may be estimated that approximately 10 per cent of ambulatory care takes place in hospital outpatient clinics.

TABLE 6

CONSULTANT-STAFFED OUT-PATIENT CLINICS STATISTICS
NUMBER OF SESSIONS AND ATTENDANCES BY SPECIALTY DURING 1983

Specialty	Sessions	Attendance		
		New	Return	Total
Cardio-Vascular	1,977	8,046	43,143	51,189
Cerebral Palsy	60	76	110	186
Dermatology	2,166	16,573	36,741	53,314
Endocrinology	1,149	3,174	23,524	26,698
Endoscopy	221	1,165	2,684	3,849
E.N.T.	4,155	30,488	47,801	78,289
Gastro-Enterology	871	4,541	15,526	20,067
Genito-Urinary	1,452	6,898	24,045	30,943
Gerontology	583	1,854	4,424	6,278
Gynaecology	4,684	22,470	43,780	66,250
Haematology	573	799	9,124	9,923
Medicine	8,085	28,857	120,476	149,333
Neurology	1,074	5,636	13,041	18,677
Neurosurgery	436	1,687	5,618	7,305
Obstetrics	7,239	53,071	212,968	266,039
Oncology	1,456	6,561	56,178	62,739
Opthalmology	6,550	29,436	79,080	108,516
Orthopaedics	4,841	37,312	117,610	154,922
Paediatrics	4,067	14,423	48,587	63,010
Plastic-Surgery	580	4,257	13,131	17,388
Psychiatry	2,483	4,902	27,084	31,986
Renal	749	1,019	8,521	9,540
Respiratory	571	1,510	7,550	9,060
Rheumatology	785	2,815	11,840	14,655
Surgery	9,415	70,784	197,302	268,086
Total	66,222	358,354	1,169,888	1,528,242

4. REMUNERATION

4.1 PRINCIPLES

Each employed person in the state pays a compulsory contribution - Pay Related Social Insurance PRSI. This is 8.5% of earnings up a to specified limit (IR£13,000 at present). A reducing scale applies to earnings above this figure). Persons paying into a pension fund may opt to pay a lower percentage (3.5%) of earnings up to the specified figure. The Health Services provide free primary (GP) cover for 38 per cent of the population in the GMS scheme, and free outpatient ambulatory care for a further 47 per cent.

The only other major health insurance scheme is a private one operated by the Voluntary Health Insurance Board which is a state sponsored, but not controlled, body. Thirty per cent (30%) of the population are covered by this insurance.

Remuneration in both the GMS and VHI schemes is largely on a fee for service basis. Per capita remuneration is unusual but occurs occasionally in some industrial medical situations with physicians in occupational medicine. Remuneration for consultants providing outpatient ambulatory care is paid on a sessional (3 hours) basis. At present the salary is approximately IR£2,000 per weekly session worked.

The GMS scheme also provides a rural practice allowance (IR£2,130 per annum in 1984) for doctors who live and provide a service in a centre with a population of less than 500 and where there is no town with a population of 1,500 or more within a three mile radius of that centre.

4.2 SURVEILLANCE

In the GMS scheme the Medical Officer, of their Payments Board, investigates claims submitted by a doctor which appear to indicate that the rate of attendance has been excessive or appear in any other way unreasonable, or where prescribing appears to be abnormal. If the Medical Officer decides, he may refer the circumstances to an investigating group of three doctors, from agreed panels appointed by the Minister of Health, the Irish Medical Organisation (IMO) and the relevant Health Board. This group may warn, make a deduction from remuneration or refer the case to a committee to consider termination of the doctor's contract. The doctor concerned may appeal to a further committee nominated by the Minister and the IMO. In 1982 nine doctors were investigated for matters related to claims.

In the VHI scheme the patient pays the doctor after each treatment episode, receipts and pharmacists dockets are submitted to the Board at the end of each year.

Under the terms of the Hospital Consultants 'Common Contract' Consultants may be monitored on their provision of services. To date this is unusual.

5. STRUCTURE OF PATIENTS

5.1 INSURANCE STATUS

There are three categories of eligibility for health services benefits in Ireland:-

CATEGORY I — Families are covered by the GMS 'Medical Card' scheme. This group comprises 38 per cent, the lowest income group.

CATEGORY II — Families with income below an annually specified limit (IR £13,500 for 1985). This group comprises 47 per cent of the population.

CATEGORY III — Families whose income is above the specified limit. This group comprises of 15 per cent of the population.

The services provided are:-

CATEGORY I — Full range of health services without charge.

CATEGORY II — Free maintenance in hospital public wards.
Free specialist services outpatient services in public clinics.
GP maternity and infant care services.

CATEGORY III — Free maintenance in hospital public wards.
Free specialist services at public outpatient clinics.

The VHI scheme, while mainly providing cover for costs of private accommodation in hospitals and consultant fees, also provides outpatient benefits up to IR£1,400 per annum. This covers GP fees, costs of investigations etc. The first IR£146 however, in any one year is not covered. Premiums for VHI are tax deductable.

From the above figures it is seen that, while most citizens are covered for hospital care including outpatients, only 68 per cent (38 per cent GMS, 30 per cent VHI) are insured for GP primary care.

5.2 MORBIDITY SPECTRUM

It is difficult to estimate the morbidity spectrum relating to primary/ambulatory care. This is because the medical nature of the consultation is not recorded except in a general sense in hospital outpatient clinics. Some indications of general morbidity may be obtained by perusal of Tables 6,7,8,9 and much other relevant information in reference (1).

5.3 TREATMENT SPECTRUM

Comparison of Table 6 with Table 7 gives some indication of the treatment spectrum.

TABLE 7 NUMBER OF CONSULTATIONS WITH GMS DOCTOR (1984)

HEALTH BOARD	SURGERY	DOMICILLARY	TOTAL
EASTERN	1,623,508	424,738	2,048,246
MIDLAND	473,403	93,622	567,025
MID-WESTERN	533,739	106,481	640,220
NORTH EASTERN	620,555	115,340	735,895
NORTH WESTERN	559,701	143,898	703,599
SOUTH EASTERN	766,875	189,772	956,647
WESTERN	894,215	176,614	1,070,829
SOUTHERN	987,607	239,133	1,226,740
TOTAL	6,159,603	1,489,598	7,949,201

TABLE 8

LONG-TERM ILLNESS SCHEME — NUMBER OF PERSONS AVAILING BY MEDICAL CONDITION, 1981 AND 1982

Condition	1981	1982
Mental Handicap	2,242	2,386
Mental illness (children only)	131	152
Phenylketonuria (P.K.U.)	157	251
Cystic Fibrosis	591	649
Spina Bifida/Hydrocephalus	1,135	995
Haemophilia	147	162
Cerebral Palsy	705	772
Epilepsy	9,879	10,504
Diabetes	15,384	16,294
Multiple Sclerosis	990	837
Muscular Dystrophies	154	175
Parkinsonism	993	1,067
Acute Leukaemia (children only)	262	314
Total	32,780	34,558

6. ACCOUNTING

6.1 REQUIREMENTS

The documentation required for claims are GMS 'two part' forms. These require details of the time of consultation, and whether a) in the surgery and b) domicillary visits, which also require information on the distance travelled as different fees apply for each category.

Double basic surgery fees apply to certain procedures: removal of cysts, suturing, ECG, draining hydroceles, family planning. These are claimed for on a separate procedure form.

Diagnosis or therapy codes are not in use at present. There are no restrictions but claims are monitored and visiting rates prescription forms analysed. Claims to the VHI are made by presentation of receipts for consultation and treatment. There is no charge for hospital outpatient consultations unless the patient is non eligible in which case he is liable for the consultants fee.

6.2 TIME AND STRUCTURE

GMS claims are submitted on a monthly basis. The treatment period is based on each consultation. Eligibility is authenticated in the GMS service by a 'Medical Card'. A Hospital Card or a VHI number is required in the ambulatory care outpatient services.

6.3 PROCESSING

Claims are processed on a monthly basis by the General Medical Services Payments Board. VHI claims for GP or private outpatient services are made on an annual basis.

7. MEDICAL DOCUMENTATION

All doctors are required to document the notifiable infectious diseases of patients under their care. (Table 9) This attracts a small fee. The National Drugs Advisory Board also encourages all doctors to document actual or possible drug interactions.

8. GOVERNMENT, NON-GOVERNMENT ORGANISATIONS AND PROFESSIONAL BODIES

The Department of Health,
Custom House,
Dublin 1.

The General Medical Services
Payments Board,
Raven House,
Finglas, Dublin 11.

The Post Graduate Medical
and Dental Board,
Corrigan House,
Dublin 2.

The Central Statistics Office,
Earlsfort Tce,
Dublin 2.

The Irish Medical Organisation,
10, Fitzwilliam Square,
Dublin 2.

The Irish College of General
Practitioners,
Corrigan House, Dublin 2.

TABLE 9 **CASES OF INFECTIOUS DISEASES NOTIFIED**

	1982	1983
Acute anterior poliomyelitis	1	–
Acute encephalitis	4	7
Acute viral meningitis	54	191
Anthrax	–	–
Bacillary dysentery	143	212
Bacterial meningitis (including meningococcal septicaemia)	124	141
Brucellosis	159	126
Cholera	–	–
Diphtheria	–	–
Food poisoning (bacterial other than salmonella)	68	83
Gastro enteritis (when contracted by children under 2 years of age)	2,404	2,987
Infectious mononucleosis	55	196
Influenzal pneumonia	6	76
Legionnaires Disease	2	2
Leptospirosis	4	14
Malaria	33	17
Measles	1,897	6,180
Ornithosis	–	–
Plague	–	–
Rabies	–	–
Rubella	166	2,395
Salmonellosis (other than typhoid or paratyphoid)	175	205
Smallpox	–	–
Tetanus	–	–
Tuberculosis	975	n.a.
Typhoid and Paratyphoid	4	4
Typhus	–	–
Venereal diseases	n.a.	n.a.
Viral haemorrhagic diseases (including lassa fever and marburg disease)	–	–
Viral hepatitis: Type A	184	237
Type B	26	53
Type unspecified	1,066	1,192
Whooping cough	1,073	1,728
Yellow fever	–	–

n.a.: not available.

9. STATUS OF COMPUTER SUPPORT

9.1 TYPES

At present only three systems are being actively offered in Ireland. Each has been developed by local software and marketing companies in cooperation with one or two General Practitioner's designed to suit the local market. All three systems are built on data base filing structures and have an acceptable range of hardware options.

The software in each system supports all the usually expected features of a professional GP system for example administrative features such as Accounts, Billing, Income Expenditure, Appointments as well as more clinical applications, Medical History, Drugs/Interactions, Age/Sex, clinical risk registers, prescriptions and automatic recall letters etc. These features are known to be cost effective in many environments. All also supply facilities relevant to the GMS scheme. Major hardware vendors have not yet shown great interest in the GP market. Some have had occasional episodes of activity.

In the hospital outpatient area, the two major companies involved in hospital computing in Ireland, SMS and McAuto, have or are in the process of implementing outpatient clinic management systems in several hospitals.

9.2 PENETRATION

To date the use of computers in General Practice is rare. There are possibly less than a dozen 'professional' systems in operation all supplied by the three active vendors. One of the vendors has recently come to an arrangement, with a pharmaceutical marketing company to supply very heavily subsidised systems to selected General Practitioners, 20 to date. It is hoped that this boost may lead to greater interest in computerization.

9.3 PROBLEMS

The current problems in Ireland with regard to the introduction of computers in general practice are not related to procedures of admission or accreditation, which are non existent, nor to legal obstacles. Data protection laws and regulations are still at the discussion stage. Health computing professionals voluntarily abide by the Council of Europe guidelines.

The major problems in effect lie with user 'resistance, bias, apathy or antagonism' to quote one salesman. The reasons for this are obviously multifactorial, however among them are:-

a) The structure of Primary Health Care. The fee for service payment based on a consultation period with no requirement of detailed clinical documentation.

b) Only 50 per cent of doctors maintain appointments systems and 30 per cent make some effort to maintain age/sex registers. (3)

c) The number of group practices in Ireland is very small.

d) Forty two (42) per cent of doctors do not employ clerical staff and a further 32 per cent employ only part time clerical staff. (3)

e) No positive incentives have been offered from the Department of Health or Health Boards either to encourage group practice or to computerize.

f) The computer in the present payment system is unlikely to be of economic benefit to the doctor. For example cervical smear testing, vaccination schedules and other procedures do not yield increased income.

10. TRENDS AND FUTURE DEVELOPMENTS

It is unlikely that the computer will play a major part in the area of Primary care in Ireland unless the General Practitioner receives greater benefit from computerization than is achieved at present. Thus the notable contribution to epidemiology and morbidity and standards of patient care which the computer has been shown to make are unlikely to occur in Ireland unless positive incentives are introduced by Central Government. Although one Health Board has recently sponsored a system on a trial basis in a selected practice. These facts have been recognised in the Report of the Working Party on the General Medical Service. (8) Finally it is also possible that the pharmaceutical industry under threat from the move to generic prescribing, may increase the level of sponsorship and cause computing in General Practice to become more fashionable.

I should like to thank Marie O'Brien for typing, and John Gloster, Vincent Pippet and Reginald Spelman for much helpful advice.

11 REFERENCES

(1) Statistical Information relevant to the Health Services (1984).
The Stationary Office, Molesworth Street, Dublin 2.

(2) Report of the General Medical Services (Payments) Board 1984.
Raven House, Finglas, Dublin 11.

(3) Oliver, B., Meagher, N., Cole M. (1984).
The present state of General Practice in the Republic of Ireland. Modern Medicine of Ireland (Supplement).

(4) O. Sé, L., Reilly, W.B., Hurley, Mary, (1982).
Survey of doctors in Community Medicine I. Med. J. 75, 74 - 78.

(5) The Post Graduate Medical and Dental Board First Report 1980 - 1985.
Corrigan House, Dublin 2.

(6) Irish Medical Times (1985) 19, 45. P. 9.

(7) Zimmerman J. Physician utilization of Medical Records: preliminary determinations (1978) Med Informatics 3, 27 - 35.

(8) Report of the Working Party on the General Medical Service 1984.
The Stationary Office, Molesworth Street, Dublin 2.

Primary Care Computing in the U.K.

by Dr. Norman Stoddart M.B.,B.S.

General Practitioner,Calverton, Nottingham.
I.C.I. Computer Fellow to the Royal College of General Practitioners

The functions of computer systems in use in primary care in the U.K. are dictated by the limitations of inexpensive microcomputers and the almost unique method of delivery of primary care within the National Health Service (NHS). The NHS has some similarities in Italy, and to a lesser extent, Holland and Scandinavia. Only a tiny proportion of primary care in the U.K. is delivered privately and will not be considered in this paper.

Structure of primary care

The NHS in the U.K. is under the control of the Department of Health and Social Security (DHSS). The DHSS is further divided unequally into three national areas, one for England and Wales (80% of the U.K. population), one for Scotland and one for Northern Ireland. Each national division is administered separately but in almost identical ways. For the purpose of simplicity only the situation in England and Wales is discussed in detail in this paper.

The NHS is divided into two divisions :-
(a) Hospital and Community Services
(b) Family Practitioner Services.(FPS)

It is in the division of FPS that primary care is delivered.Approximately 30% of medical graduates work in this area.

Every person in the U.K. is registered and allocated an NHS number. Identification details of each individual including NHS number, name, address and date of birth in England and Wales are held by the NHS Central Register and updated at intervals by the Population Census and Surveys. This register is at present run manually but will probably be fully computerised by 1987. Day to day administration and registration is conducted by Family Practitioner Committees (FPCs) in geographical local areas. There are 90 FPCs in England and 8 in Wales. 46 of these FPCs have computerised registration and the remainder should be computerised within two years.

Recently FPCs have been given complete autonomy from their corresponding Area Health Authority which administers the hospital and Community Health Services.

Contracting Practitioners who provide primary care have a self employed status and contract with the local FPC to provide their services. These contractors are General Medical Practitioners (GPs), Dentists, Pharmacists and Opticians.
Each individual patient is registered with a specific GP. The FPC pays a capitation fee to the GP for each patient. In return the GP provides all necessary medical primary care. This capitation fee is the same whether the patient requires no treatment or extensive treatment, except that all patients over 65 years attract a higher capitation fee and a still higher fee for those over 75 years. What is expected by necessary care is not well defined particularly in the case of anticipatory and preventive medicine.

In an attempt to encourage such extra care item of service fees are paid for night calls, PAP smears for women over 35 or those of parity 3 or more, immunisation, contraceptive services and maternity services. There is no form of peer review of the quality of this care.

The GP has open access to most x-ray and pathology facilities and it is the GP who decides when it is necessary to refer a patient for secondary care.

The GP may practice from health centres provided by local authorities in which case the rent is reimbursed by the NHS or from premises provided by the practitioner personally in which case a "nominal rent" is paid to recompense the capital outlay. Most GPs work in partnership, the average practice having three partners. There are variations from single handed to more than ten partners in a practice. Each doctor has on average 2,100 registered patients.

Ancillary staff are employed by the GP directly. 70% reimbursement of the cost of employing staff is paid by the NHS up to a maximum of two full time staff per doctor. The average practice at present employs 1,2 full time staff per doctor as either receptionist, clerks, secretaries, dispensers, nurses or practice managers. Often the local Community Health Department attaches district nurses and health visitors to the practices at no cost to the practitioner.

When treating a patient the GP can prescribe medications or appliances which are then supplied by a pharmacist of the patient's choice. In rural areas the GPs may contract to dispense themselves. Dispensing doctors claim the cost of all prescriptions, receive a dispensing fee and also receive a slightly larger capitation fee for a patient registered for such services. Prescriptions are written on standard forms and after being dispensed are processed through a single Prescription Pricing Authority (PPA) before repayments are made via the FPC to the contractors. The PPA is due to be fully computerised by 1987.

Administration links within the NHS

Department of Health and Social Security
(DHSS)

England & Wales (80% of UK population) | Scotland | Northern Ireland

Family Practitioner Services(FPS) | Hospital & Community Health

NHS Central Register | Area Health Authorities

Family Practitioner Committees(FPC) | District Health Authorities

General Medical Practitioners (24,000 in 8,000 practices) | Pharmacists (10,000) | Dentists (14,000) | Opticians (8000)

Presciption Pricing Authority(PPA)
(One central agency)

Documentation

Since 1948 all registered patients have a medical record. This is an envelope 12.5cm x 17.5cm in which letters and notes are stored. This method of recording dates back to 1912. The document is the property of the DHSS and is held by the registered GP. If the patient moves the transfer of this record is organised by the FPC(s) involved. There are no guidelines as to what recording is made, this is left to the discretion of the individual GP but some guidance is given by the Medical Defence Societies because of the medico-legal importance of such documentation. A small proportion of practices have replaced these records by A4 folders.

All claims for fee for item of service and claims for ancillary staff are made on a multitude of different forms, none suitable for computer processing. Prescription forms however are available in continuous fan-folded form for computer printing and supplied free from the FPC to the GP.

Requests for x-ray and pathology investigations are made on forms common only to the local hospital but most pathology reports are returned printed by computer.

Any adverse reaction to a drug treatment should be reported on a hand written form to the Committee of Safety of Medicines, an organisation mainly charged with surveillance of recently introduced drugs. Adverse reactions are probably grossly unreported, 50,000 reports by 20,000 doctors being made from 1972 to 1980. Recently a view data system has been tried in a few practices to encourage reporting.

Non-governmental organisations in primary care

The General Medical Services Committee is a branch of the British Medical Association and is concerned with the conditions of service for GPs.

The Royal College of General Practitioners is an academic body concerned with the quality of primary care and with education including vocational training for general practitioners.

The Joint Computer Policy Group is an advisory group with representatives from both the above two bodies together with representatives from the D.H.S.S. and the Primary Health Care Specialists Group of the British Computer Society. This body has been concerned with standards of software and computer printing prescriptions and has been the prime mover in the detailed testing of general practice computer software which is at present in progress.

Legal requirements

A recent Act of Parliament - the Data Protection Act - will require all users of computers in the U.K. who hold personal data to register by May 1986. This register will be available to public scrutiny, listing all users with details of what type of information is held, from whom it is obtained, to whom it may be divulged and to what use it will be put. Any person may request details of all information held about themselves personally in any of these data banks. Registration will also require certain standards of security. All computerised medical files will be subjected to this Act but some provision, as yet undetermined, will be made to prevent information which may not be in the patient's interest from being divulged to the patient except through a Court Order.

Vocational training

Following full registration, usually one year after graduation, a doctor must complete a further three years vocational training before being able to become a principal in general practice. One year of this is spent in general practice under the guidance of a trainer. 7.5% of general practictioners are involved in this training at any one time. Trainers, who are paid by the NHS must be approved by the Joint Committee on Postgraduate Training for General Practice. This is the only area at present subject to peer review in the FPS. The criteria for selection as trainers are enthusiasm, attendance of a training course, quality of premises and records, practice library, an age-sex register, cover when on call,team work, audit and teaching time.

Finance available for computers

At the present time the cost of purchase and maintenance of computer hardware and software has to be met in full by practices. In 1983 150 practices in a pilot scheme were provided with half price computer systems by the Department of Industry during Information Technology Year.

In Scotland one free software (GPASS) is provided by the Scottish Home and Health Department providing the practice meets the cost of the hardware also required.

Influence of the NHS system on U.K. GP Computing

The independent status of general practitioners meeting the cost of computer hardware has led to almost all GP computing being run on single terminal micro-computers. At first, from 1980, these machines were usually 8 bit with floppy discs but increasingly since 1983 have been hard discs on 16 bit machines.

In 1985 at least 530 such practices are running what has become termed the typical "office" system. Because of 70% staff reimbursement the machines are unlikely to be used to replace staff, indeed computing practices have increased their staff strength, many up to the maximum of 2 full time per doctor.

Because of the clearly identified list of patients one of the first functions has been setting up an age-sex register. It is probably this facility that has made training practices 5 times more likely to computerise than ordinary practices. Setting up the age-sex register has been much easier in areas where the FPC is already computerised. In such cases the practice list has been transferred from the FPC computer via an intermediate floppy disc to the practice computer.

Once the age-sex register is complete the organisation of preventive recall for PAP smears, immunisation etc. can be pursued efficiently increasing the item of service income of the practice. It is for this increased workload that more ancillary help, including nursing, is required. Some practices, especially those involved in teaching, add hypertension, diabetes and thyroid checks and some include all items of morbidity. Less than 20 practices have terminals in the consulting room, often attempting a more extensive record than the simple problem list. The present systems with keyboard input make such recording time consuming and tedious. The majority of systems recording problem lists use some sort of coding system, many devised by the practice themselves. Of those using published coding systems most use the RCGP classification of diseases, problems and procedures (RCGP,1984), some use ICHCPP-2(WONCA & WHO,1979 & 1983) or OXMIS (OCHP,1978), and a few are now experimenting with the new ICHC (WONCA & WHO,1986 a&b).

Prescribing

It is in this area that in the near future GP computing shows most promise. In the U.K. patients on long term medication are often issued with repeat prescriptions. These are traditionally issued on a monthly basis without the doctor seeing the patient except on infrequent occasions. Many manual systems have been developed using either inserts in the patient record or a card held by the patient's themselves listing the drugs to be taken. These lists are faithfully copied out by ancillary staff at the patient's request usually with the date recorded when issued and the printed prescriptions are then signed in batches by the doctor. Such a function is easily computerised. In such office systems there is often a practice formulary of drugs used by the practice which may include action, drug interaction and contraindications. The system allows automatic audit of prescribing,often recording the date the patient was last seen and when next due to be seen by the doctor, checks on patient compliance and warning of possible drug interactions. The need for comprehensive drug database has recently been accepted by the Information Technology Working Party of the R.C.G.P. Such a system should be compatible with the PPA. A coding system at present being considered is the Nordic Drug Code. However a knowledge base for intelligent prescribing will also be required. In the U.K. at the present time drug databases available are Martindale Online and a view data system "Treatment" produced by Klewer. A further database is also being developed by the Association of the British Pharmaceutical Industry (A.P.B.I.) None of the databases would be usable in their present form for expert prescribing but the potential is there.

With the promise soon of cheap multiterminal systems the possibility of a prescribing system used within the consultation room for all prescribing should be possible. Suggestions have been made that such systems could eliminate the paper prescription by using instead some form of plastic smart card carried by the patient. A pilot study for this has been proposed in a recent report to the DHSS (Arthur Anderson & Co. 1984).

Expert systems

Development of expert systems in the U.K. are confined to small well defined areas of medicine e.g. abdominal pain, dyspepsia, chest pain, E.C.G.analysis. None at present show signs of being able to cope with the problems in more uncertain areas in which primary care is usually conducted. In the early stages of development computerised protocols for specific disease management e.g. hypertension and diabetes are more manageable.

Present state of computing

Over 120 different softwares are being used and developed in the U.K. Almost all are "Office systems". Most of these are systems used by only one developing practice but 35 are being offered commercially.

The DHSS is soon to publish the results of detailed testing of these systems. Over 100 of these softwares applied to be tested but only 14 were able to fulfil the criteria for this testing:
(1) to be able to load an artificial databank of 10,000 patients with some details of morbidity and medication provided by the DHSS,
(2) to have had the system in at least one other practice other than the development practice for at least 6 months.

In June 1985 a questionnaire was answered by 188 practices using computers for a mean time of 2 years 3 months. The following frequency of collection of specific items of data and their use was reported to me:-

<u>Items of data</u>

Age-sex register

Name	144
Address	116
Date of birth	142
Occupation	49
Marital status	95
Name of registered doctor	128
Date registered	110

Repeat prescriptions

Printing	133
Drug interactions	42
Contraindications	24
Audit of patient	68
Audit of doctor	56
Stock control	7
Bottle labelling	21

Risk factors

Smoking	64
Alcohol	48
Parity	37

Problem list	67
(" " using coding system	63)
Record summary	80
Encounter notes	21

<u>Call & recall system used</u>

Immunisations	Measles	70
	Pertussis	70
	Dip.and/or tetanus	75
	Polio	71
	Rubella	79
	'Flu	62
PAP smear		91

Recall Clinics

Contraception	51
Wellwoman	36
Wellman	20
School leaver	15
Diabetes	37
Hypertension	42
Thyroid disease	20

Other uses

Appointments	10
Encounter notes	21
Consulting room use	16
Chronic disease protocols	21
Patients recording own history	9
Patient instructions	46
Fee claims processed	12
Accounts	26
Word processing	105
("" not integrated with files	68)
("" integrated with patients files	37)
View data	26

The future

It is likely that primary health care computer systems in the U.K. will for some time remain dominated by the NHS. Networking will be particularly feasible between FPCs, GPs, Pharmacists and the PPA, plans for this being already well advanced. Methods of networking between primary and secondary care are at present more nebulous.

Software will probably develop in a less haphazard fashion following the formal testing of the present softwares. The foundations for setting up knowledge bases in primary care have still to be laid down and it is at this level that systems will have common ground on an international scale, but the problems of achieving this seem immense.

Conclusions

Since 1980 the use of simple office systems have increased from a mere handful of users to 530 practices. The tasks performed by these machines are directed by the NHS method of delivering primary health. Advances are hindered by cost and unsophisticated single terminal hardware. The foundations for networking are being laid but remain mainly in the field of practice management. Little progress has been made so far in clinical applications beyond age-sex registers for preventive care and repeat medication. Computer assisted prescribing offers a useful first task for the advance in clinical applications.

References

Arthur Andersen & Co. (1984) Report of a Study of Family Practitioner Services Administration and the Use of Computers Commissioned by DHSS and Welsh Office, London, Arthur Andersen.

Oxford Community Health Project (1978)OXMIS Problem Codes for Primary Care. Oxford . OXMIS Publications

Royal College of General Practitioners (1984) Classification of Diseases, Problems and Procedures 1984, Occasional Paper 26, London, R.C.G.P.

WONCA and WHO (1979) An International Classification of the Health Problems of Primary Care. (ICHPPC-2). Oxford, Oxford University Press.

WONCA (1983) ICHPPC-2 Defined. Inclusion Criteria for the Use of the Rubrics of the International Classification of Health Problems in Primary Care. Oxford. Oxford University Press.

WONCA and WHO (1986a) International Classification of Primary Care (ICPC). Oxford, Oxford University Press. In press.

WONCA and WHO (1986b) International Classification of Primary Care: Process. (IC-Process-PC). Oxford, Oxford University Press. In press.

Further reading.

Sheldon M and Stoddart N. (1985) Trends in General Practice Computing. London. Royal College of General Practitioners

PRIMARY HEALTH CARE IN FINLAND

Yrjö Jokinen

Computing Centre, University of Kuopio, P.O. Box 6,
SF-70211 Kuopio, Finland

INTRODUCTION

Health care has traditionally been the responsibility of the community in Finland. The legislation of health care was thoroughly renovated in 1972 giving more emphasis on primary care. The municipalities are now responsible for the primary care and the municipal health center is the functional unit providing the basic health services for the population. Private practice has importance in towns, but in rural areas, covering the main part of the country, virtually all health care is given by municipal health centers.

The municipalities are also responsible for the hospital care. Municipal health centers often have their own hospitals, which usually do not give advanced services. Specialist level services are provided by so-called central hospitals. Administratively, the country is divided into 21 central hospital districts, formed by federations of municipalities. Five of the central hospitals are university hospitals. The state and private institutions provide only 4 % and 5 % respectively of all hospital beds in the country.

The State supports the municipalities by reimbursing over 50 % of all expenses of health care and also supports part of the private hospitals economically.

INSTITUTIONS SUPPLYING PRIMARY CARE SERVICES

Primary health care is organized in Finland on the basis of regional responsibility. Each of the communities has a health center of its own or they have established one jointly with the neighbouring communities. There are 213 health centers in the country. The size of population covered by one health center varies from 10.000 to 150.000. The city of Helsinki is an exception.

The health center is responsible for the comprehensive primary health care including dental care, children care, maternity care, occupational health and also environmental health. They have also hospital wards headed by general practitioners mainly for elderly or chronically ill patients. Some of the health centers in larger cities have also hospitals headed by specialists. On the average there are 4 beds/1.000 people in health centers. For comparison, there are 12 beds/1.000 people in other hospitals including the mental hospitals.

The number of employees in various professional groups in health centers in 1983 was the following:

physicians	2.850
dentists	1.680
nurses	5.400
public health nurses	4.200

other nursing personnel	16.280
other personnel	11.780.

For comparison, the number of physicians in hospitals in Finland in 1983 was 3.770 when total number of working physicians in the country was 9.800. The total number of dentists working in Finland was 3.500.

All personnel in health centers receives a monthly salary.

In larger cities primary care services are also given by the private group practices. Physicians in private practice are often specialists.

EXPENDITURES IN PRIMARY HEALTH CARE

The expenditures in health centers divided between the different parties were in 1983:

government	1.043	Million	DMK
communities	905	"	"
patients	148	"	"
health insurance	21	"	"
other sources	107	"	"
------			
total	2.224	"	",

which means 460 DMK/per capita/year on the average of which a person paid 30 DMK by himself.
53 % of the money is spent for ambulatory care and 47 % for the hospitals in health centers.

For comparison, total health care expenditure in Finland in 1982 was 7.640 Million DMK which is 6.9 % of GNP and 1.575 DMK per capita.

STRUCTURE OF THE POPULATION AND CATCHMENT AREAS

The structure of the population in Finland in 1982 was:

0 - 14 years	20 %
15 - 64 years	68 %
over 64 years	12 %.

The total population in 1982 was 4.845.000.

Practically all people in Finland can receive the basic primary health care. Only 2 % of vacancies in health centers were open in 1984. In rural areas there is no alternative local health care system but a patient can visit any of the providers working in the health center. In the cities, people can also visit private physicians. This option is usually taken when a specialist's services are needed.

Occupational health system was renovated in the beginning of this decade. By the end of March 1983 every employer was obliged to arrange an occupational health service for all employees. Smaller enterprises have made contracts with local health center or private group practices. Larger companies have occupational health departments of their own.

STRUCTURE OF THE PRACTICES

A health center is generally decentralized both on regional and functional basis. There are usually several health stations where a patient can visit. Dental clinics are generally located in separate buildings in different regional centers. The laboratories and x-ray departments are often located in the main health station but some of their activities like collecting the samples are also decentralized.

Because people are free to choose the health station and/or the provider, they usually go to the nearest one. This may be a different station depending whether they stay at home or whether they go to work.

The health care providers work usually full-time in the health center but e.g. a specialist in radiology may have a part-time contract.

The private group practices are generally located in downtown areas or in larger regional centers. Laboratories and x-ray departments are generally in the same building. Most often physicians work only part-time, e.g. only once a week, in a group practice having their full-time job somewhere else, e.g. in a hospital. Thus a great number of physicians may work in a group practice in a large city.

In 1983, 8.7 million visits were made to health centers and 2.8 million visits to privat group practices.

REMUNERATION AND HEALTH INSURANCE

A patient pays only a nominal fee when visiting a health center. The same is true also for the hospital services.

There is also a general health insurance in Finland which covers 50% of the costs for drugs and for the visits to private practitioners. If a patient has a chronic disease, he may apply a 100 % refunding for the drugs.

The patient receives also a daily allowance during his sick leave starting on the 7th day from the onset of the leave. In 95 % of the cases a patient receives a full decompensation from the 8th day to the 90th day. From the 90th day to 300th day the payment is somewhat smaller. Mothers receive the same allowance for their leave before and after childbirth which is 300 days. If the patient has no income he gets the minimum allowance which is 15 DMK/day.

The fees used in private practice are agreed upon in annual negotiations between the National Bord of Health and the Medical Association in Finland.

The National Social Security Institution, which is responsible for the practical execution of the health insurance has local committees, whose duty is to review the applications for refunds. Statements or certificates given by physicians are reviewed more carefully by the expert physicians of the committee if the full retirement on medical reasons or a 100 % refunding is applied for drugs. No other formal procedures are used routinely for surveillance.

ACCOUNTING AND REPORTING

National Board of Health has defined procedures for the hospitals, health centers as well as for the private practices and laboratories to report on the activities. Some of these reports are used to justify the reimbursement to the communities, others are for health statistics and for planning purposes at the various levels of the health care organization. National Board of Health receives information e.g. about every hospital admission and discharge including the diagnoses. This reporting has no direct economical implications.

Health centers and hospitals have, however, several data collection and reporting procedures running which are used e.g. to divide the costs between the member communities. Data is also collected about every occupational health service in order to be able to bill the corresponding employer.

PROBLEMS IN DATA PROCESSING IN PRIMARY HEALTH CARE

The health centers are relatively complex organization which are decentralized both on regional and functional basis. This creates problems in communication between various units.

The coordination of various activities, administration of the health center and planning of the activities as well as reporting to various parties requires more and more manual work. Sometimes it is not possible to obtain the information about the past activities at all because the need was not anticipated in due time.

The private group practices do not have all the responsibilities of health centers. Because of that some of the data processing problems are not as prominent. They have, however, all the problems of accounting and billing for the services.

One of the problems seems to be that the transfer of information between the health centers and private group practices is practically non-existent. Also the information exchange between primary and secondary or tertiary health care is often not satisfactory.

STATUS OF THE COMPUTER SUPPORT IN PRIMARY CARE IN FINLAND

The first set of guidelines or policy for computer application in health care was defined by a few working groups in 1972/73. The objectives and aims set in 1973 have been met long ago. Another working group was established in 1984 to create the new guidelines up to the year 1990. This work has not yet been completed.

These guidelines do not impose any official obligations for the communities. Furthermore, their main emphasis lies in data processing in hospitals.

The National Board of Health has a small staff in its technical department whose duty is to coordinate all EDP-related activities. The health centers and the private group practices even more so, may quite independently make their own decisions about data processing. The situation is not yet too heterogeneous mainly because there are not too many alternatives available for health centers and because the health centers do not have too much money to make hasty decisions.

There are two major products used in primary health care. The more simple system developed by the State Computing Center is used in about 100 installations for collection of administrative data, reporting and recently also for patient scheduling. The other one, called FINSTAR, is more extensive including a complete medical record subsystem. It is described more extensively elsewhere in this book.

Private group practices use often various computer systems for book keeping, accounts receivable and other applications alike. Some of them have elaborate systems for clinical laboratory. The systems for medical record or systems for data communication do not seem to have as high priority as in health centers.

There is no specific legislation for data security in Finland. Such a law has been under preparation for a couple of years now. At present, the laws and other regulations which deal with data security and integrity are spread to many sources and their application in a modern data processing environment is not easy.

TRENDS AND FUTURE DEVELOPMENTS

Integration between the information systems of health centers and hospitals seems to be a more and more important topic in the discussions about the future development. There are both technical difficulties as well as administrative difficulties.

If the coming new data law takes a very restrictive form, it may significantly hamper the pursuits for better integration.

The possibilities of creating large medical databases could be used for individual health education as part of home and self care has created also some interest. The necessary technology may find its way to homes in future.

The use of AI and expert systems in primary care fascinates only few people at the present. It may require not only more advanced technology but also a new generation of health care providers before it is more generally accepted.

The Swedish Health-Care System

H. Peterson, A. Leimanis.

Hälso- och sjukvårdsförvaltningen, P O Box 9099
S-102 72 Stockholm, Sweden.

0. Introduction

In Sweden most of the health-care is provided by the County Councils. There are 23 County Councils and three independent cities and they are semi-independent from the Ministry of Health and Social Affairs.

1. Structure of Primary Care

1.1 Supply, Institutions

In Sweden, Primary Health-Care is defined as the out-patient care which takes place outside the hospitals at Primary Health-Care Centers owned by the County Councils. They are usually open only during office hours. In the same building, there are also specific consulting rooms for district nurses, home care, child welfare and maternity welfare. The Primary Health-Care Centers are located in the areas where people live, but a few are situated in business districts. 53% of the out-patient visits are to Primary Health-Care and 47% to the Out-Patient Departments in the hospitals.

In Stockholm County with a population of 1.5 million inhabitants, there are 4 million visits a year to health-care provided by the County Council and 1.25 million to private physicians of which the majority are specialists. The situation in the country is that there are very few private physicians outside the four largest cities.

There are very few specialists working at the Primary Health-Care Centers. To see a specialist the patient usually has to be referred to a hospital.

1.2 Personnel

1.2.1 Physicians

The number of physicians in primary health-care is 3.400 and in the hospitals 9.000. The total number of physicians is 20.700 in the whole country.

1.2.2 Other personnel

At the Primary Health-Care Centers there are also a number of nurses, practical nurses, therapists of different kinds and secretaries and receptionists. The number varies very much but there are usually three nurses, two practical nurses, one secretary and one therapist for every physician and one receptionist for every two physicians.

1.3 Expenditures

Sweden uses 11% of the Gross National Product (GNP) on health-care. 90% of the expenditure is channeled through the County Councils. The rest comes from the National Health Insurance directly to the private physicians on a fee basis for services rendered.

The income of the physicians varies from Sw Cr 175.000 - 350.000 per year for those who are employees of the County Councils. The income for the private physicians varies from Sw Cr 300.000 - 450.000 per year.

2. Structure of Population and Catchment Areas

The population in Sweden is concentrated into three areas: Stockholm, Gothenburg and Malmoe regions. Nearly 20% of the population is to be found in the Stockholm area. These three regions contain more than 35% of the population. In the northern half of Sweden there are only about 15% of the population.

Sweden is divided into seven Health-Care Regions, each of them containing a medical faculty and a university hospital. As each County Council is independent, there have to be agreements e.g. how to share costs for specialized care.

Each County is divided into two to five Health-Care Districts, and these in a number of Primary Health-Care Areas. These are then divided into catchment areas containing 2 - 6.000 inhabitants.

A treatment team is responsible for this population. A Primary Health-Care Center can consist of one to six treatment teams, and one or several specialists can be working there as well. The psychiatric care is organized in the same way.

The patients are asked initially to approach their Primary Health-Care Center for treatment. As the resources are limited, there can be difficulties in getting access to another Primary Health-Care Center. For emergency treatment, the patient can be treated at any health-care institution. To be treated in a hospital or by a specialist, a referral is usually needed.

3. Structure of Practices

Most private practices are run by specialists, and only in the larger cities there are a few group practices and these are run by a number of physicians, all of different specialities. There are only four small private hospitals in the country, and these are all owned by foundations.

Almost all private physicians are organized in "Service companies for private physicians" and they own a part of their practice by holding shares and are mostly employees of the company on a fee basis for services rendered.

4. Remuneration

In Sweden all inhabitants are compulsory members of the National Health Insurance System. There are no fees as the money comes from the Government by taxation of the population.

In private practice a fixed amount of the physician's fee is refunded from the system directly to the physician. The amount depends upon which measures were necessary. The patient pays the remainder of the fee directly to the physician. As the money that comes from the National Health Insurance does not cover the cost, it is up to every physician to review the costs of the practice.

In the official health-care system the patient pays a fixed amount of 50 Sw Cr for a visit. In this sum all tests, examinations and consultations necessary are included. The County Councils are refunded from the National Health Insurance on a per capita basis. This income is only 9% of the costs and the remainder is covered by county tax money.

There is no surveillance plan or agreed procedure for paer-review. These studies are ad-hoc investigations. Within the different County Councils there are different methods of surveying the cost for every procedure and also cost per diagnosis.

5. Structure of Patients

5.1 Insurance Status

All Swedes are mandatory members of the National Health Insurance System. Very few have private Health Insurance.

5.2 Morbidity Spectrum

The number of acute visits is 32% of all out-patient visits. A large number of these take place at the emergency of the Primary Health-Care Centers. The rest is patients who can be received the same day in the ordinary way. The number of chronically ill patients especially with diabetes and hypertension are in majority. The total number of contacts in the country is 19.6 million a year or 2.3 per inhabitant.

6. Accounting

There is no accounting at all for treatment given by the County Council. The patient pays Sw Cr 50:- for every visit up to 15 for a calendar year. There after all treatment is free.

For a visit to a private physician the patient pays according to the procedures and examinations performed. The physician is reimbursed from the National Health Insurance System according to procedure codes. There is one form for every visit to be filled in. These forms are sent monthly and the content is the name of the physician and the patient, the date or dates of the visits, the procedure codes and the sum of money according to a grouping of procedures in four groups. For each group there is a fixed amount. This sum is negotiated once a year between the Private Physicians' Association and the National Health Insurance.

7. Medical Documentation

The only thing mandatory to record after a visit is symptoms or reason for the visit and treatment and other kinds of action taken.

8. Status of Computer Support in the Country

The types of computer systems available range from systems taking care of the mandatory administrative and economical information to systems covering the complete medical record. A number of translated and modified Costar systems are in use. The systems are to be found only in the public sector. The number of Primary Health-Care Centers with a complete information system is not more than 5-6. The total number of Centers is around 790, whereof 690 have more than one physician. About half the number of Centers have some kind of computer support.

In the private sector there is only one Center with a complete support. All the others have manual procedures but the information collected is centrally processed to produce statistics and calculate the refund for each physician.

There are no specific problems for primary health-care except transfer of information from the hospitals about patients who are completing their treatment in primary health-care. The problem is how much of the hospital information should be transferred and how. As a lot of the information is available on line in the hospital, the Primary Health-Care Center wants to be directly connected. For laboratory results, this is possible today but the other parts of the medical record are not available even if they are stored in a computer system. The system with discharge notes is usually too slow to be of any use.

9. Trends and Future Developments

The trends are to computerize the medical record and make it available where and when it is needed. A new legislation will make this possible if the patient agrees to the transfer of the information. This is applicable only in the public sector. In the private sector, the physicians will keep their record and they will not be a part of a computer network.

There is a development going on aiming at computer support for the Primary Health-Care Center as a unit. This system can communicate with all laboratory computers and the hospital information system at the hospitals to which they are sending their patients.

INFORMATION SYSTEM IN DOCTOR'S OFFICE IN JAPAN

Y. Yanagita, M.D.

Tokyo Maternity Clinic, 1-20-8, Sendagaya, Shibuya-ku, Tokyo, Japan 151

INTRODUCTION

Every country has its own medical system, and it has been influenced by the government policy, by the history and also by the economy of that country. In Japan, there are two remarkable characteristics concerning the practice of medicine, which has much to do with the information system in doctor's office.

MEDICAL MILIEU IN JAPANESE DOCTOR'S OFFICE

Firstly, 99 % of the Japanese population are under government social health plan and the costs for each treatment are set by the government.

Whether the professor of surgery who has 25 years of experience performs the gastrectomy or the young surgeon who has just finished his internship does it, the charge to the patient is the same. The experience and skillfulness of the physicians are not taken into account in the government social health plan.
For example, when the young unexperienced surgeon develops complications during surgery, he needs longer times to finish the operation. As the charge to the patient is in proportion to the medicine and surgical material he has used, he may charge more money to the patient than the professor does.

This is a kind of joke, but it is theoretically true. So every patient would like to go to the university or university affiliated large hospitals, so that a doctor at these clinics has to see more than 100 patients in one morning at his clinic.

The 'form' to print the item of treatment or medicine to get the money from the government social health fund is called "RECEPT" and activities involved to make "RECEPT" are called "RECEPT MAKING".

Secondary, a characteristic of the Japanese medical system is, not like that of the United States, every hospital has its own large outpatient department.

Thirdly, there are quite a few small clinics in Japan. They are, with some exceptions, not well equipped and the physicians there are not well educated from the standpoint of continuing medical education. The nursing staffs at those clinics are always short and most of them are also not very well educated from the standpoint of modern medicine.

Japanese physicians are trying to utilize the computer to solve the daily problems at practice.

Outpatient departments may occupy 1/3 to 1/4 of the area of a large hospital; there computers are increasingly used (Fig. 1 and 2).

Fig 1 Numbers of Computer in Hospital in Japan

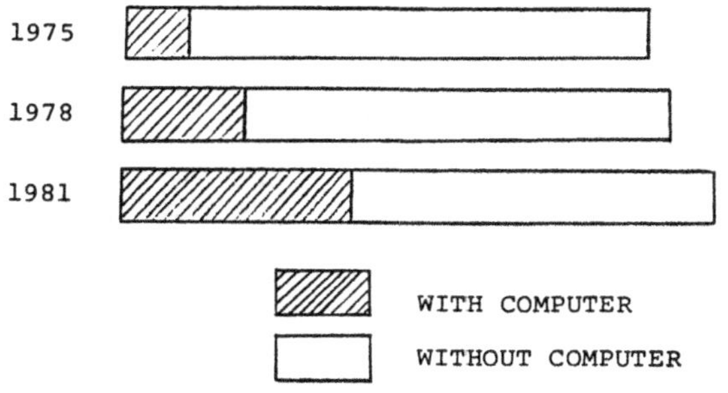

Fig 2 Numbers of Computer in Hospital in Japan

BEDS	1975	1978	1881
20 - 49	8.6 %	14.0 %	28.6 %
50 - 99	11.2 %	20.9 %	38.9 %
100 - 299	15.5 %	27.2 %	49.3 %
300 - 499	26.0 %	37.7 %	58.3 %
500 -	35.5 %	52.1 %	73.1 %
AVERAGE	13.4 %	22.8 %	41.7 %

Because of the wide-spread government social health plan, policy for treatment of certain sickness is strictly limited and preplanned. So computers are most frequently used at the cashing department.

In 1983, 24% of the "RECEPTS" are made by computer. "RECEPT" is a 'form' to print items of treatment to get the money from the government social health fund after the patient has been treated (Fig. 3 and 4).

Fig 3 "Recept Making" by Computer (Clinic and Hospital)

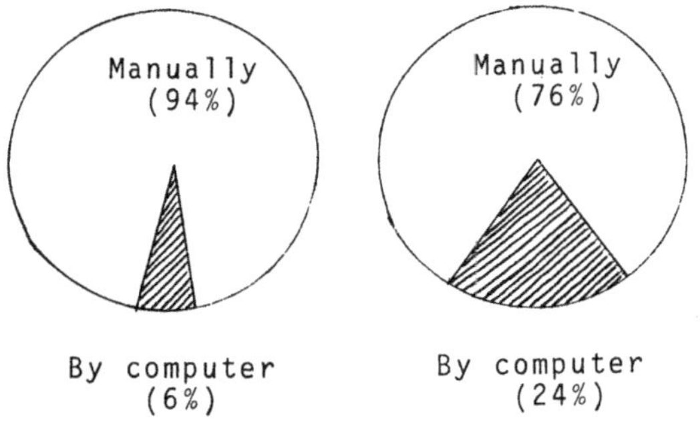

Fig 4 "Recept Making" by Computer Clinic

MONTH YEAR	No. of Doctors	Drs. that use Comp.	%
May 1980	77,026	4,932	6.4
May 1981	77,917	6,406	8.2
May 1982	78,386	7,907	10.1
May 1983	78,347	9,857	12.6
May 1984	78,546	12,260	15.6

Depending on the policy of local medical associations in Japan, the use of the computer in the different parts of Japan varies from 9.0% in Akita to 25.6% in Nagano. This is illustrated in Fig. 5.

Fig 5 "Recept Making" by Computer

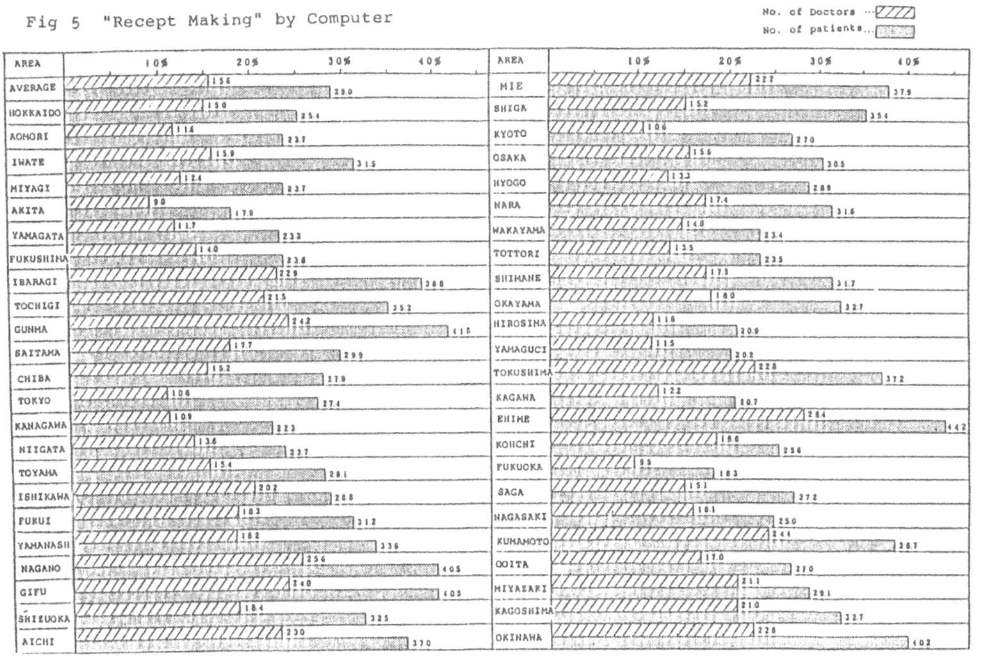

FOUR MAJOR DIFFICULTIES IN INTRODUCING PRACTICAL INFORMATION SYSTEMS IN JAPAN

There are 4 major problems so far in Japan for introducing computer in practice. Firstly, Japanese use Chinese character but there are more than 3,000 fundamental 'characters' in Chinese writing characters, comparing with 25 characters in English, so that inputting a Chinese character into the computer is a very troublesome matter and the efficiency of inputting data is very low.
Secondary, people in the United States and in Europe get accustomed to use the typewriter from their childhood contrary to Japanese people.
Thirdly, the communication lines were all owned and operated by the government until recently and the cost to use the line has been very high.
Fourthly, the government puts strict regulations to connect the computer to telephone lines.

JAPAN MEDICAL ASSOCIATION'S POLICY FOR DOCTOR'S OFFICE INFORMATION SYSTEM

In 1985, the Japanese Medical Association (JAMA) published policy statements on computers. Most members of the Japanese Medical Association are practicing physicians and about 60% of the practitioners are enrolled in this association.

The JAMA established a committee to discuss the use of computers in medical practice in Japan. Their main subject is to set a standard 'form' to produce a "RECEPT". Besides this subject, JAMA investigated the actual use of computer in local areas. The computers are used in 28 prefectures of 47 prefectures in Japan for emergency patient transfer system. Fig. 6 shows the one in the Nagoya area as an example.

Fig. 6 Emergency Patient Transfer System in Nagoya area.
This system is very satisfactorily working.

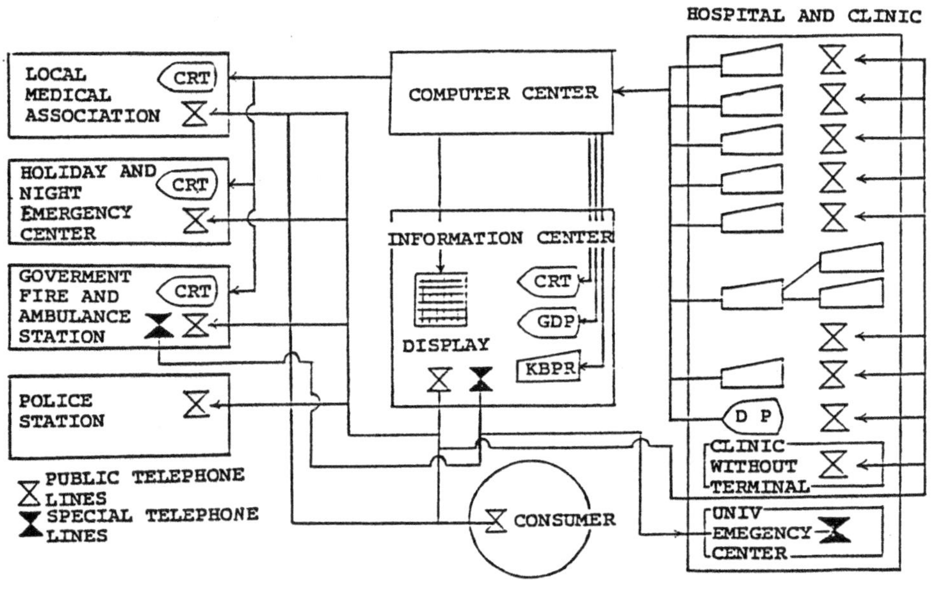

But this does not mean that all physicians in this 28 prefectures have their own computers. And some part of these information is transmitted by telephones. Computer analysis of ECG through telephone lines from the doctor's office are now used in 23 prefectures in Japan.
Local area medical information systems for residents are established in many local areas and most of them use computers.
Also medical professional information service systems such as epidemiology surveillance, drug side effect surveillance, etc. are set up.

The computer systems mentioned above are working well but the hospitals or clinics which actually use these systems are very limited and actually a very small number of Japanese physicians can use these information, just because very few doctor's own computers and also they don't know how to connect the computer to telephone lines. So except for making the "RECEPT", very few doctors use computer in daily practice.

EXEMPLES OF COMPUTER USE IN DOCTOR'S OFFICE BESIDE "RECEPT" MAKING

Computer minded internists and dieticians use hand-held computer for calculation of calories and balanced intake of vitamines, minerals, and iron as well as fat, protein and carbon hydrate. This is very helpful for instruction to diabetics and obese patients.

Obstetricians and gynecologists use computer to calculate the gestational weeks and EDC from ultrasound examination (Fig. 7). They also use microcomputer for estimation of fetal weight and its growth.

Fig 7 Ultrasound Calculation of Gestational Week. Lines show, from left to right, standard growth curves for GS, CRL, BPD and FL. Black squares show growth of this fetus.

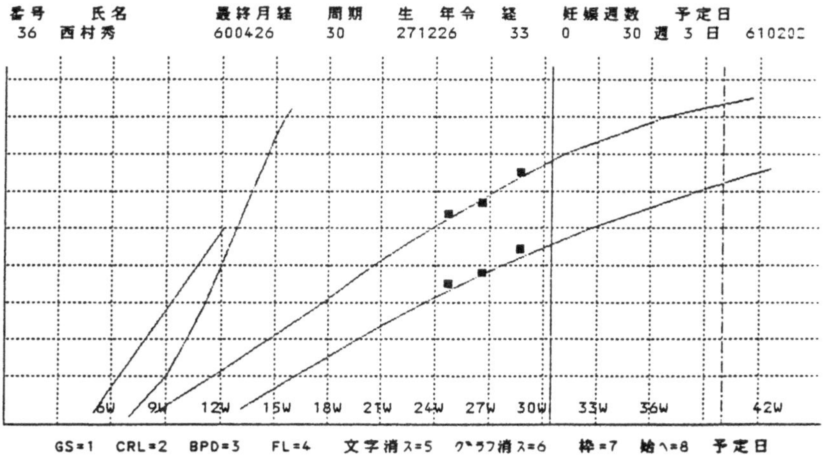

SUMMARY

1. In Japanese doctor's office, computers are mainly used to 'make recepts' to claim money from the government social health funds.

2. Local area networks for 'emergency patient tranfer systems' are being built under the sponsorship of Japanese Medical Association (JAMA) and they are functioning well.

3. Computer minded Japanese physicians use microcomputer at doctor's office for making database or as diagnostic support. But the total number of computers used for this purpose is very limited.

4. Information transfer through the public telephone lines are just made possible by the change of Japanese Communication Regulation Law. So except very rare cases no doctors have established a system to get information through the public telephone lines so far.

5. But in near future many physicians working at the clinic will get diagnostic help through their computers connected to the public telephone lines.

REFERENCES

N. KAIHARA, (1985) Medical Care and Computer, Nippon Hyoron Sya, p. 66.

Y. YANAGITA, (1985) Medical Care and Computer, Nippon Hyoron Sya, p. 56

Y. YANAGITA, (1985) Fully Portable Perinatal Database System Using Hand-held Microcomputer with Itemized Keyboard, Archives of Gynecology, p. 237, 34.

STRUCTURE OF PRIMARY HEALTH CARE IN THE NETHERLANDS

C.A. de Geus en A. Hasman

INTRODUCTION

In this paper the structure of the Dutch Primary Health Care Services will be discussed. The Dutch Government stimulates new developments in this area to ameliorate the quality of care in the Health Care System as a whole and to lower expenditures.

1. STRUCTURE OF PRIMARY CARE

1.1 Supply and institutions

In the Netherlands primary health care is supplied by the first echelon of the Dutch health care system This system is functionally divided into echelons according to a 1974 policy proposal, as follows (Tiddens 1984):

Basic echelon	(Extramural and preventive treatment)
First echelon	(Extramural and curative facilities)
Second echelon	(Specialized facilities for outpatient and inpatient care)
Third echelon	(Facilities for permanent and long term intramural and extramural care).

The echelons aren't clearly defined as there are areas of overlap. Division into echelons is still commonly accepted as useful.

A fundamental feature of the first echelon is its easy accessability. By general practitioners, district nurses, midwives, pharmacists and dentists this is guaranteed 24 hours a day and at acceptable distances for everybody. Special regulations are in force in the weekends and to some extent during evening and night.

Physiotherapists are also in the first echelon. Access to them and to the pharmacists is indirect after referral by the general practitioner (GP).

The ease of access is for some persons and in some situations relative if we take into account differences in financial barriers.

Another discipline in the first echelon is social work. It is practised as an independent job, in health centres or in mental health care teams.
GPs, nurses and social workers are more or less involved in the treatment of mental health care problems. Other professionals active in this field are psychiatrists, psychologists, psychotherapists and psychosocial workers. About 100 different institutions provide ambulatory mental health care. Coordination of organisations and attunement of the various areas of work to each other is placed increasingly in the hands of the regional institutes for ambulatory mental health care (RIAGG). The professionals mentioned are reckoned among the providers in the first echelon so far as they are attached to the RIAGG-institutes.
With the exception of psychiatrists in the RIAGGs no specialists are

active in the first echelon. Their domain is in the hospitals or institutes for permanent and long term care in the second respectively third echelon. To get across the boundary line between the first and the second echelon people need to be referred by the GP and to enter the hospital. The GP occupies a 'gate-keeper function'. Hospital-based first aid facilities however have a low barrier and their use requires referral by the GP afterwards. This situation causes controversy as expensive specialized care is not always indicated.
General practice, physiotherapy and midwifery are mostly private enterprise. Nurses, social workers and members of mental health care teams are in service of their employers, respectively the National Cross Association, a 170 institutions of social work, jointed in the JOINT, and the Dutch Association for Non-clinical Mental Health Care.
Family Welfare work is practiced in the first echelon by certificated professionals and laymen under their guidance, many of them in part time functions.
The Ministry of Welfare, Health and Culture is in charge of management and control of the health care system as a whole and of its employees.

1.2 Personnel

The number of GPs has increased from 4.809 in 1975 to 5.900 in 1985 (CBS, Statistisch Zakboek 1985). This means 2.450 inhabitants per GP. TABLE 1 presents figures of Primary Health Care providers, physicians in basic, 2nd and 3rd echelon and other physicians (this category includes GPs and specialists in training, physicians in scientific education, in research institutes, nursing homes and military services.

Table 1. Primary health care providers except those active in ambulatory mental health care and medical social work; numbers of physicians in second, third and basic echelon, and others (1985)

5.900	General Practitioners		
	. 5.900		
	. 10.796	Medical Specialists	
	. 1.787	Public Health Physicians	
	. 12.707	other active physicians	

	31.185	physicians	
4.415	Nurses (fulltime equivalents)		
1.013	Nursing aids		
6.805	Dentists		
1.800	Pharmacists		
950	Midwives	|-	3.700 settled
7.900	Physiotherapists	-|	
		|-	4.200 f.t.e. fulfilled by partimers as cooperators of the settled ones

Practice ancillaries, usually certificated, are responsible for administrative tasks, act as receptionists, perform simple laboratory work and assist with first aid.

1.3 Expenditures

The costs of health care rise considerably as a function of time. The costs in 1980 amounted to 8,34% and in 1984 to 8,6% of the gross national product at market prices. Total cost has risen in the years 1982, 1983 and 1984 from about 32.000 via 33.000 to about 34.000 millions of Dutch guilders. The amount increases to 40.833 mln if social and psychosocial services are included. Throughout these years expenditures for institutions for intramural health care, extramural health care and other health care are constantly 59%, 36% and 5% of the total cost respectively.
So the cost of extramural health care in 1982 amounted to fl.11.575 mln.
The money is spent for general practice and suppliers of medicines, dressings, prosthetic appliances etc. (9020 mln), for institutions for social health care (1905 mln) and for other institutions like ambulance (650 mln) (Vademecum voor Gezondheidsstatistiek, 1984). The share of general practice in the total cost for health care reduced from 5,1% in 1977 to 4,4% in 1983.

The GP with a norm practice receives a norm income, which is fixed on a rather high level of the pay scale for civil servants. A norm practice, which is a model for calculation, comprises 1750 sickness fund patients and 750 private patients. The gross norm income amounted to fl.220.000,- in 1983. About the half is remuneration, the other half comprises practice expenses and contribution for pension. By deduction of taxes the net income is again about a half of the remuneration and can be estimated at over fl.50.000,-.

2. STRUCTURE OF POPULATION AND CATCHMENT AREAS

The Netherlands are a densily populated country with about 14,5 mln. inhabitants (Nederlandse Statistiek van de Bevolking, mei 1985). In 1981 the average age of Dutch men and Dutch women was respectively 33.4 years and 35.8 years. The average age is rising steadily in recent years, because of a remarkable reduction of infant mortality since 1950 (CBS Statistical Yearbooks, 1950-1980) and an increasing life expectancy for all ages. For those born in 1982 the mean life expectance is calculated to be 72.7 years for men and 79.4 years for women (CBS, Statistisch Zakboek, 1984). Never before has life expectancy been on that level. The percentage of 65 and over in the population has increased from 11.5 in 1980 to 12 in 1985 (Tiddens, 1984; CBS, Maandstatistiek van de Bevolking, 1985). It is expected that this percentage will rise further in future. A particular growth of the percentage of old aged is foreseen.

The death rate in 1975 was 8.32 per 1.000 (CBS, Statistical Yearbook), in 1984 it was 9.1/1.000 for men and 7.6/1.000 for women (CBS, Month Statistics).

Table 2 presents leading causes of death in 1980.

Table 2. Estimated death rates per 100.000 population for leading causes of death, 1980, the Netherlands.
Source: Statistical Yearbook

Diseases of the circulatory system	362.2
Neoplasms	220.3
Diseases of the respiratory system	49.5
External causes of injury and poisoning	43.1
Symptoms, signs and ill defined conditions	37.8
Diseases of the digestive system	27.7

Death rates by traffic accidents descended remarkably over a period of ten years (1973-1983) from 23.5 to 13.5 per 100.000.
Table 3 shows leading diagnoses in general practice in percentages of the total number of diagnoses (IMS, Diagnose Analyse uit de praktijk van Huisartsen, 1976).

Table 3. The five leading diagnoses in percentages of the total number of diagnoses in general practice (1976)

Family planning	4.81
Benign hypertension	4.47
Symptomatic coughs	2.62
Bronchitis	2.39
Nervousness	2.12

Table 4 presents the top 10 chronic diseases in general practice (Voorn,Th.B. 1983)

Table 4. The top ten known affections in general practice per 1.000 patients (1978)

	Men		Women
Obesity	58	Obesity	118
Hypertension	33	Hypertension	77
Nervous complaints	31	Nervous complaints	70
Chron. bronchitis	28	Varices	67
Arthrosis	22	Arthrosis	42
Hardness of hearing	22	Hardness of hearing	20
Angina pectoris	15	Diabetes mellitus	17
Myocardial infarction	14	Myogeneratio Cordis	13
Varices	12	Angina Pectoris	13
Diabetes mellitus	11	Constitutional Eczema	11

Table 5 presents the top 10 reasons for encounter as registered in 8 practices (Registration Network Family Practices, Rijksuniversiteit Limburg, 1985).

Table 5. The top 10 reasons for encounter in a registration of 10.000 encounters in 8 practices (1983)

Cough	6,2 %
Hypertension uncomplicated	3,2 %
Fever	2,9 %
Contraceptive medication	2,5 %
Symptoms/ complaints throat	2,3 %
Symptoms/ complaints back	1,9 %
Rash	1,8 %
Headache	1,8 %
Local abdominal pain	1,7 %
Ear pain	1,7 %
	26,0 %

The Dutch health care system offers free access to the first echelon (GP, dentist, midwife, nurse, social worker). The patient registers himself as a patient of the GP of his own choice. He is free to change. The norm practice is 2.500 people. Measures are taken and in preparation to reduce practices with over 2.500 people in favour of small practices and young doctors.

The Cross Organizations serve 75% of the total population, who become members of a local organization by paying a contribution. Nurses and nursing assistents provide nursing at home, inclusive aid for GP or midwife, mother and newborn in case of home delivery, given by specially trained nurses. Articles for home nursing are on loan. Care, guidance and information for diseased, invalided and elderly people is offered. Services of a dietician are in a number of cases available. The majority of nurses are stationed in district offices, a small minority in health centres. A district encompasses 30.000 - 50.000 people, 9 - 15 nurses and a chief-nurse. In a district there are several offices. The catchment population of nurses is on the average 3.200 - 3.400 people, but there are exceptions on both sides (NIVEL, De eerste lijn in kaart gebracht, 1985). Social workers have a catchment population of on the average 8.000 people.

3 STRUCTURE OF PRACTICES AND THEIR USAGE

3.1 Types

The GPs play a central role in the Dutch health care system. They fulfill their job in different settings. A clear shift to teamwork can be observed - fig 1 - (NIVEL, Statistische gegevens over huisartsen en verloskundigen, 1985).

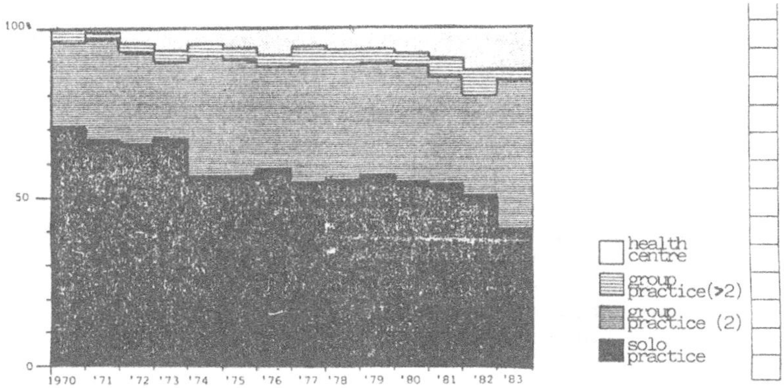

Fig. 1. Type of practice of GPs that have settled in the period 1970 - 1983.

There are 4 types of practice: single practice with one GP, duo practice with two, group practice with three or more GPs and health centres. Health centres encompass at least 2 GPs, a nurse and a social worker. Other first echelon disciplines may also be represented. The numbers of GPs in different types of practices are presented in table 6.

Table 6. Number of GPs in different types of practices (abs. and %) per 1-1-1984

	Single	Duo	Group	Health Centre	Total
Abs.	3.490	1.547	305	410	5.752
%	61	27	5	7	100

Government stimulates the quantitative growth of teamwork by means of financial regulations and special forms of subsidy. Health centres and their GPs are in engagement of foundations which are their employer. As for other professionals there are contracts between the foundation and themselves or their organizations, that attach them.

Usage. Table 7 reports data about consultations with a GP in 1 year (CBS Maandbericht Gezondheidsstatistiek, Sept. 1985).

Table 7. Consultations with a GP in 1 year 1983/1984

% persons with consultations	71,4 (10 - 14 yr. - 52,2 ≥ 75 yr. - 82,6)
Number of consultations per person in the population	3,4 (10 - 14 yr. - 1,7 ≥ 75 yr. - 5,9)
Number of consultations per person with consultation	4,8 (10 - 14 yr. - 3,2 ≥ 75 yr. - 7,1)

4. REMUNERATION

4.1 Principles

The GP receives payment for patient care in two ways. He receives a capitation fee for patients who are insured by a sickness fund. The sickness fund pays the GP a fixed amount per registered patient every three months, irrespective of whether the patient requires his services or not The total per capita fee is paid for a maximum of 1.600 registered patients. For 1.601 and over the pension contribution drops away and the contribution for the costs decreases at once.

Private patients are treated on a fee-for-service basis, the GP being paid by the patient himself. The patient will get restitution from his health assurance and he is insofar insured for this form of care.
Fee-for-service charges are fixed in tariffs for consultations at the doctor's office and at home, irrespective of the extent of health care activities or the time spent per encounter.

4.2 Surveillance

Because the capitation fee for sickfund patients is very simple, no surveillance is needed. The number of registered patients on fixed dates decides the fee paid to the GP.
Private patients get bills by the quarter of the year. Dates of doctor's visits and the names of family members that are treated, are reported on the bills. Reporting of these data is requested by the insurance companies. It is more and more unusual to leave reporting data, even if this is not mandatory. The GP is constrained in his prescription of drugs. Only drugs accepted by the sickness fund may be prescribed. The fund checks prescriptions after receiving them from the pharmacist. The GP therefore can only be corrected afterwards. There are no sanctions, only private interviews on the initiative of the sickness funds. Patients have to pay a certain amount of money per prescription themselves.

5. STRUCTURE OF PATIENTS

5.1 Insurance status

Patients are insured either by a sickness fund (66,6%) or privately (33,4%). The number of people without any health care insurance is neglectable, but a proportion of private patients is insured only for specialist treatment and hospital care (Stichting KLOZ, informatie systeem gezondheidszorg, Jaarboek 1984).
For employees and their families insurance by a sickness fund is compulsary when their income is below the wage limit, as determined by the Sickness Allowance Act. Insurance by a sickness fund as a facility for other people, whose income does not exceed the wage limit, will be lifted up this year (1985). Special regulations are in force for employees in public service (collective insurance; fixed own risk as a percentage of health care costs and fee for service basis) and for military men.
High risks like serious and prolonged illness and disability are insured by a national insurance, regulated by the Exceptional Medical Expenses Act. Sickness funds and admitted private health insurances are charged with the execution of the mentioned Act.

5.2 Morbidity Spectrum

This is discussed before in chapter 2.

5.3 Treatment Spectrum

Data about the number of consultations with a GP are presented previously in table 7. Data about specialist-treatment-cards are published in the Yearbook LISZ 1983 by VNZ, Zeist 1984, as a product of the National Information System on Sickness funds of the Netherlands. The deliverance by GPs of specialist-treatment-cards in 1983 amounted to 507/1.000. Top five were cards for oculist (108), surgeon (70), internal medicine specialist (54), specialist for diseases of nose, throat and ear (42) and gynaecologist/obstetrician (39).
Sickness funds send at intervals anonymised lists to the GPs to inform them about the numbers of specialist-treatment-cards, delivered by them and their colleagues in the past period. No signifant differences are demonstrable in this respect between single practices and group practices or health centers.

6. ACCOUNTING

6.1 Requirements

Mandatory documentation requirements are discussed in paragraph 4.2. Specialist-treatment cards are administrative; no medical information is recorded. The GP who refers a patient gives a letter with relevant information for the specialist and a circumscribed request as to his intervention. It's under discussion whether the envelope should be open or not.
Physiotherapist treatment cards and inquiries for supplies such as large quantities of dressings need to report a reason or motivation for referral c.q. inquiry. No codes, only descriptions are used.

6.2 Time and structure

Time and structure of accounting are discussed in paragraph 4 as this information in the context of that paragraph was basic for explaining remuneration and its surveillance.

7. MEDICAL DOCUMENTATION

There is no obligation for GPs to document medical information, although every GP keeps record of his patients. The most popular form of documentation is the so-called 'green card'. A number of GPs make their notes with application of the SOAP-scheme. They keep a problem oriented record on patients. A relatively small number uses preprinted forms in family-maps for problem oriented recording.

8. GOVERNMENTAL AND NON-GOVERNMENTAL ORGANIZATIONS AND PROFESSIONAL BODIES

In the Netherlands the Ministry of Welfare, Public Health and Culture is responsible for health care. Health care, provided by academic institutions is under control of the Ministry of Education. The Universities are charged with postgraduate training. It must be executed in cooperation with professional bodies. For that purpose an organization was instituted in 1985 to structure the cooperation. It has uniprofessional sections and mixed professional committees. The Royal Dutch Association of Medicine has its National Organizations for GPs (LHV), specialists (LSV) and physicians in public service (LAD). The Association serves the interests of its members on an international, national and regional/local level. About 85% of the GPs is a member. The Dutch College of General Practitioners (NHG) with about 50% of the GPs as a member is primarily a body that is concerned with scientific issues.

9. STATUS OF COMPUTER SUPPORT IN THE COUNTRY

9.1 Types

The percentage of GPs, owning a computer system has been estimated to be less than 2% at the moment. The use of the computer was mainly for financial and administrative purposes. One system, installed in the pharmacy, is used for medication surveillance. To this end, some GPs have a terminal, connected to the system by telephone, in their office.
A number of computer systems were developed by GPs themselves. In order to guarantee, that systems,that should be bought by GPs, were able to communicate and in order to guarantee that terminology etc. would be standardised a government subsidized project was started in 1979. This project was terminated in 1985 and resulted in functional and technical specifications for computer systems for general practitioners. These results have been used by a committee of the above mentioned organizations LHV and NHG to specify the minimum requirements that systems for general practitioners should fulfill. Vendors must have their systems hallmarked before the committee will advise GPs, that the system is of sufficient quality to be bought.
The functional specifications concern the set-up of the screens, the contents of the modules, out of which the system should be built up etc.
The hallmarking procedure is still under discussion but will be established within a few months.

9.2 Penetration

Since the hallmarking procedure is still under discussion no hallmarked system is yet on the market. A number of computer vendors and software houses have expressed their willingness to develop systems for general practitioners on the basis of the earlier mentioned specifications. However a small number of systems, developed for financial administrative purposes were already in the market. Recently, a system developed in cooperation with a GP was introduced in the region of Gorinchem and supported by the sick fund in that region. Also in other places systems are being developed, supported by sickness funds. A few systems are being developed at the moment in cooperation with universities.
An information campaign is set up at the moment with the aim to reach about 20% of the 5.800 GPs in the country in order to inform them about the status and expectations of computerization of primary care. After having followed such a program the GPs should be able to take the correct decisions concerning the introduction of a computer system into their practices.
A government subsidized project will be started, that will investigate the added value of computerised methods for the GP.

9.3 Problems

No specific problems are anticipated. There still is no data privacy law in force in the Netherlands. The systems have to fulfill the customary requirements for optimal datasecurity. Since the financial administration is rather simple, the penetration of computers into the private practice is slow. The purchase of a computer system is still expensive and the advantages are not always very clear. There is still a relative large group of GPs having their own pharmacy (± 20%). It can be expected that the introduction of computer systems in these practices will be faster.

10. TRENDS

The introduction of computer systems into the private practice will have important consequences. At the moment only scarce data are available about the complaints of patients, visiting the GP. For policy making more insight into the actual demand is important. Several studies have been performed about referral patterns of GPs. With the help of a computerized system the GP can compare his own functioning with that of his colleagues (self audit). With the help of videotex faculties post-graduate education can be facilitated. Expert systems and decision analytic programs can be introduced into private practice. By collecting data from a larger group of practices epidemiologic data, worthwile in the GP practice can be developed. Medication surveillance can be more easily performed.
The information exchange between the workers of the first echelon and between these workers and the hospital also becomes feasible. A number of feasibility studies are executed in the Netherlands to obtain an idea about what information is transferred between the various participants in the health care system. In this respect also the value of the use of the smart card, containing the data of the patients, is under study.
Implementation of the International Classification for Primary Care has been started in a number of practices. Awaiting its authorization by the WHO, the professional bodies tend to accept the ICPC in the GP-information system. By several GP research groups in our country it is adopted. A computerized Network of Family Practices, affiliated with the State University of Limburg, with a nineteen doctors, trained in the appliance of the ICPC is prepared to generate data for research purposes.

REFERENCES

Tiddens HA, (1984). Health Services in the Netherlands. In Raffel MW Comparative Health Systems, the Pennsylvania State University Press, University Park and London.
Statistisch Zakboek CBS (1985). Geregistreerde werkzame geneeskundigen, p. 63.
Vademecum Gezondheidsstatistiek Nederland (1984). Financial data about health care. p.178.
Maandstatistiek van de bevolking, CBS (sept. 1985). Population of the Netherlands by marital status and sex per five years age group, January 1st 1985. p.18.
Statistisch zakboek CBS (1984). Gemiddeld aantal te verwachten levensjaren naar leeftijd en geslacht. Life-expectance. p.41.
IMS, Nederland BV, Den Haag. Tabel 11, p. 26.
Voorn TB (1983). Chronische ziekten in de huisartspraktijk, wetenschappelijke uitgeverij BUNGE, Utrecht.

De eerstelijn in kaart gebracht, NIVEL (1985). Wijkverpleegkundigen. Kaart 21 p.41, Kaart 22 p.42.

Statistische gegevens per 1 januari 1984 over huisartsen, aspirant huisartsen en verloskundigen NIVEL (1985). Tabel 6, p.17.

Maandbericht Gezondheidsstatistiek CBS (Sept. 1985). Consultationss with a GP in 1 year, by age group, sex and type of insurance, 1983/1984. Number of consultations per person in the population. Number of consultations per person with consultation. Tabel 2, p.16.

KISG84; Stichting KLOZ Informatiesysteem Gezondheidszorg, Jaarboek 1984. Tabel 2, p.11. Tabel 12, p.21.

Jaarboek Landelijk Informatie Systeem Ziekenfondsen '83. Tabel 3.4 p.42; p.43.

Address of the authors:

Dept. of Medical Informatics and Statistics
Rijksuniversiteit Limburg
POB 616
NL-6200 MD Maastricht

THE BELGIAN PRIMARY CARE SYSTEM

Dr. W. Peumans - I.C. SYSTEMS
G. Verwilghensingel 4 -B-3500 HASSELT.

1. Structure of Primary Care - Personnel - Expenditures

In Belgium primary care is delivered by general practitioners (+/- 13.000), specialists (+/- 4300 =1/3 of all specialists), dentists (+/- 5.800), pharmacists (10.363, - 5.543 officinas), physiotherapists (12.400), midwives (3.442), and visiting nurses (+/- 4000).

Expenditures:

Belgium spends less than 6 % of its GNP on health care, +/- 260 billion BF in 1984.

EXPENDITURES FOR HEALTH-CARE AS A % OF G.N.P.

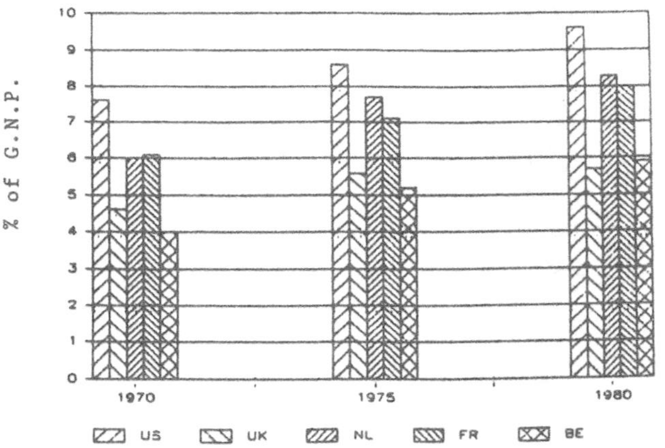

SOURCE: OECD. PARIS 1983.

EXPENDITURES FOR HEALTH-CARE PROCEDURES

	1970	1975	1981
Index all procedures	100	155	208
Index office visits G.P.	100	125	170
Index office visits specialists	100	131	165
Index radiology	100		234
Index clinical pathology	100		279
Index nuclear medicine		100	677

Source : RIZIV Brussel 1984

EVOLUTION OF MEDICAL AND PARAMEDICAL PERSONNEL
per 10.000 inhabitants

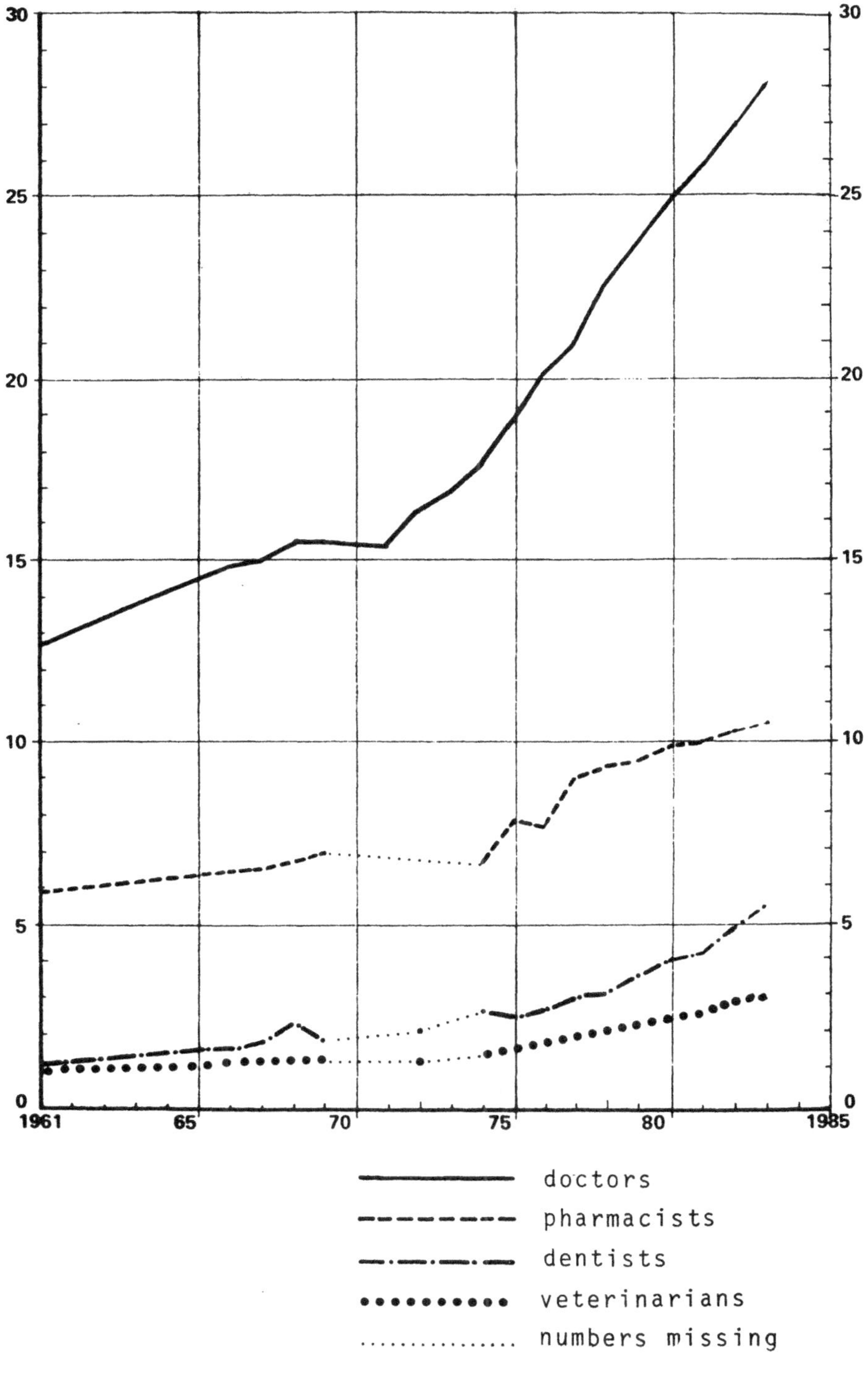

MEDICAL CONSUMPTION 1970-1981 DOCTORS AND SICKFUND AFFILIATES

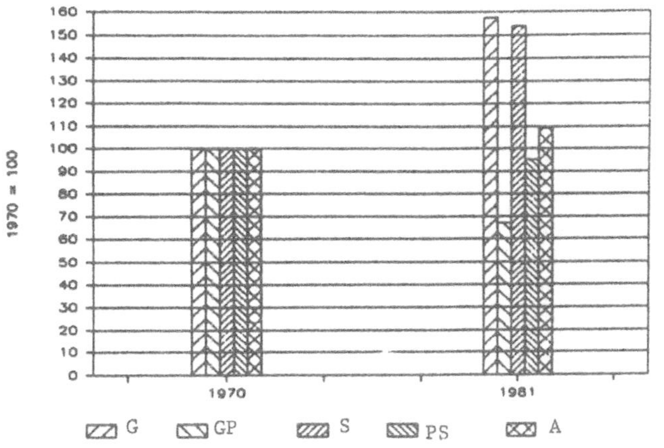

G = general practitioners
GP Proceed / G.P.
S = specialists
PS = Proc. / Spec.
A = Affiliates
P : Procedures

SOURCE: HET MEDISCH EN PARAMEDISCH AANBOD IN BELGIE, BRUSSEL 1983.

Doctor's income dramatically decreased due to slower growth of the budget for health-care, which is a result of the overall economic crisis and due to the increase of the number of practicing physicians.
In Belgium there is no numerus clausus for medical students although it was asked for by doctors unions for almost 20 years, but the successive governments refused to take any appropriate measures claiming a numerus clausus to be anti-democratic.
Meanwhile the underemployed and unemployed young physicians feel no comfort at all in being sacrificed on the altar of this principle which in their opinion serves only as a cover for the politicians' lack of courage.

DISTRIBUTION OF DOCTORS

	in practice			no practice			total		
	men	women	total	men	wom.	total	men	women	total
General Practitioners	10.830	2.155	12.985	1.042	438	1.480	11.872	2.593	14.465
Junior Specialists	2.178	899	3.077	-	-	-	2.178	899	3.077
Specialists	9.230	1.804	11.034	173	79	252	9.403	1.883	11.286
TOTAL	22.238	4.858	27.096	1.215	517	1.732	23.453	5.375	28.828

C.I.V.-C.T.I. Situation: 31/12/1984

AGE AND SEX LIST OF DOCTORS

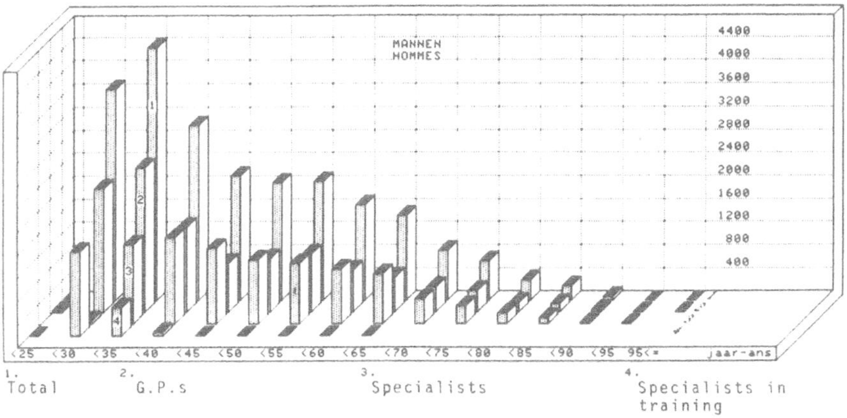

2. The structure of the Belgian population

The structure of the Belgian population (+/- 9.850.000- 10% immigrants) is changing as in most western countries towards a smaller number of births and an increase in the number of elderly people.
Morbidity shows a shift towards chronic diseases in all segments of the population.
Mortality statistics indicate the same trends as in other European countries.
There is a slight decrease in cardiovascular-mortality and a slight increase in tumour-mortality.
Patients have free access to both general practitioners and specialists.
They also can go and see several physicians as often as they wish.
Since most physicians respect the "agreement" fees and the sickfunds reimburse almost immediately 75 to 100 % of the physicians' fees to the patients there is no punishment for an abuse of this privilege.

3. Structure of practices

There are two kinds of general practitioners in Belgium - those who go in general practice immediately after medical school and those who had supplementary post-graduate courses for 200 hours.The latter have a higher fee for office visits and for house-calls.
In general practice single practices prevail (> 90 %), group practices number less than 5 %, partnerships +/- 5 %.
Group practices between G.P.s and different specialists are exceptional.

+/- 550 outpatient clinics outside the hospital exist.
Many of them are run by the sickfunds. But even there the specialists work as independent solo practitioners except in a few clinics and hospitals of the socialist sickfund and in university-hospitals where physicians share the income or what is left after management takes its part.

AGE AND SEX DISTRIBUTION OF POPULATION

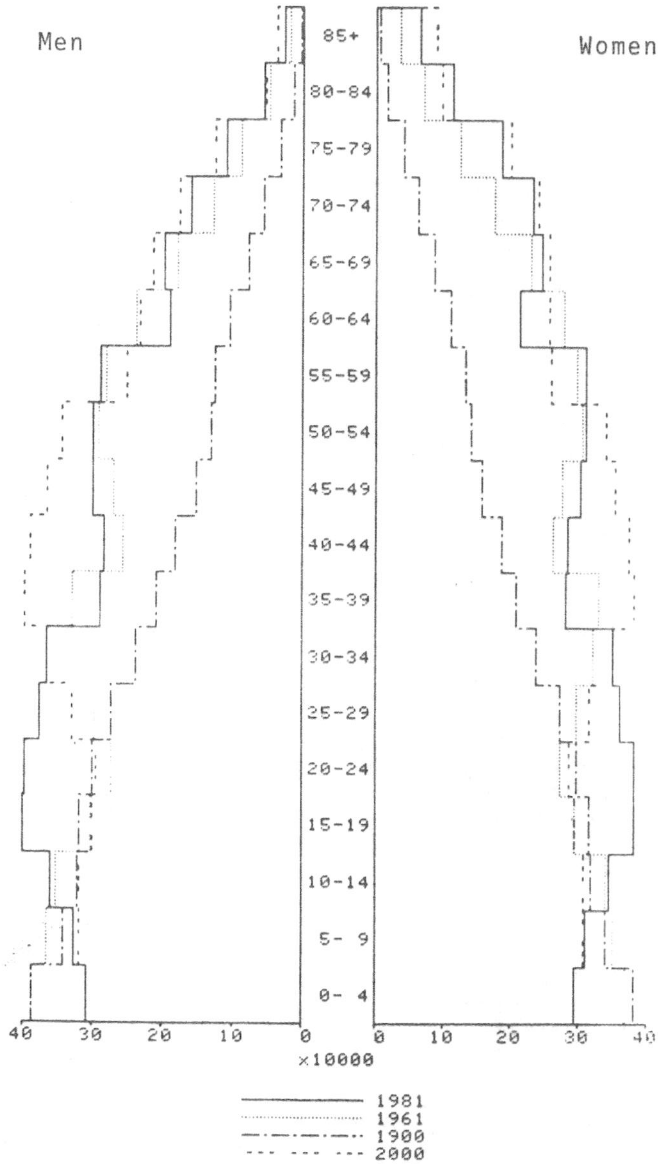

INTERNATIONAL COMPARISONS PERINATAL DEATH

°/oo births

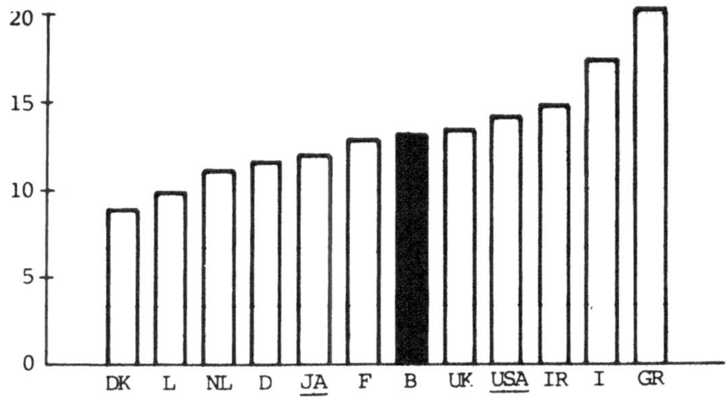

°/oo live birth

NEONATAL DEATH

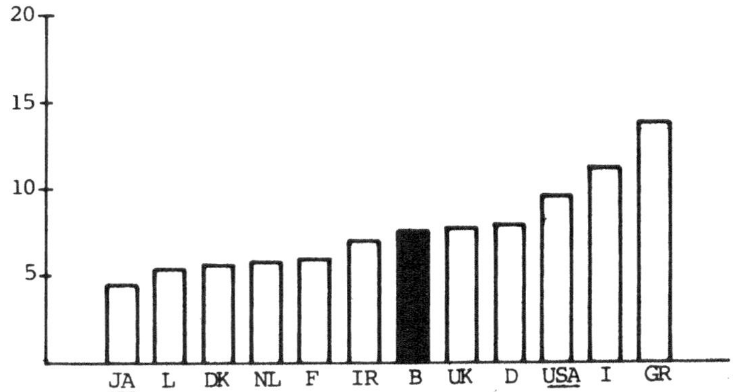

°/oo live birth

INFANT DEATH

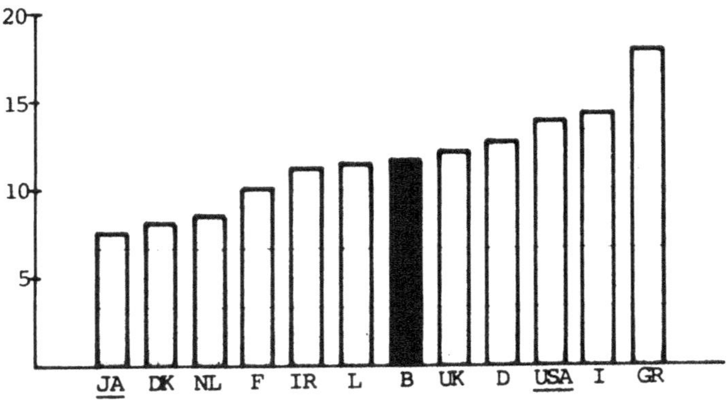

These facts indicate the preference of the people for a "colloque singulier" when looking for medical care. A reason for this and other attitudes of the Belgian people lies in the deep-rooted suspicion of the people towards authority. What is now called "Belgium" has been an occupied country for ages.
Suspicion towards the authorities has not completely disappeared when the occupying forces did.
This also could explain the poor compliance of the doctors with prescriptions for recording epidemiological data.

4. Remuneration

Belgium has compulsory health insurance which covers 100% of the population for major risks and more than 95% for small risks via the sickfunds. Doctors' unions and sickfunds negotiate an "agreement" on the fees for item of service. This agreement has to be approved by the Minister of Social Affairs.
Private insurance by commercial companies is exceptional but tends to increase lately for additional coverage of hospital costs which are not always totally reimbursed.
The remuneration is based on fee for service. Even when the physicians in group practices are paid as employees, the lumpsum comes from fee for service payments.
A few experiments launched by the sickfunds in order to promote prepaid group practice seem to lack viability.

Surveillance:

Surveillance of the ethical behavior of physicians is done by the "Orde der Geneesheren". The "Orde der Geneesheren" is a public organism created by law in order to serve both as a disciplinary court and as a legislative body for medical ethical behavior. In each province 12 physicians are elected by their peers every 6 years. They are assisted by a magistrate appointed by the king, and are qualified to judge complaints from patients, employers or from other physicians. The complaints range from excessive fees to lack of care or other misbehavior.
Administrative control is done by a control committee of physicians appointed by the National Institute for Health and Disability Insurance (RIZIV). This control committee can suspend a physician from reimbursement of his fees by the sickfunds.
If this committee feels that besides the administrative failures the accused physician acted unethically a complaint will be brought to the disciplinary court of the "Orde".
This implicates that a doctor can be punished twice once by the control committee or by the courts and a second time by his peers at the disciplinary court and this time for ethical reasons.

Doctor's income:

The income of the Belgian physician has been severely eroded as a result of the above mentioned factors.
Especially the G.P.s are affected - and very angry about it - since it became known that the working costs of the sickfunds are 150% of the total fees for general practitioners.
Compared to other professional groups physicians in general and G.P.s in particular incurred a greater decline in income.
In comparison with other western countries Belgian doctors have also much lower income.
Notwithstanding all this the quality of health-care remains at the level of other European countries. We all hope it will stay that way.

	DOCTOR's INCOME G.P.'s	Specialists
1974	1.011.895	1.354.111
1975	1.130.237	1.523.813
1977	1.332.746	1.856.513
1978	1.483.808	2.048.167
1980	1.623.461	2.262.295
1981	1.600.507	2.103.674

5. Structure of patients

Only a small percentage of the population is not covered for small risks. Major risks are covered for nearly 100 % of the population. Morbidity in general practice shows a similar picture as in other European countries.
Treatment: except for a few, the G.P.s can prescribe all drugs. Formerly reimbursement was quite high, but government intervened in order to reduce costs both by cutting the list of reimbursed drugs, and by demanding a personal contribution for reimbursed drugs.
Major surgery e.g. heart surgery is covered as a major risk. Even organ transplants are reimbursed, provided there is a donor.

6. Accounting

Requirements: reimbursement is 75 % for small risks, 100 % for major risks.
Orphans, widows, retired people and the disabled are reimbursed 100 % for all medical care (except for office visits and house-calls where a contribution of 6 to 10% is charged). Reimbursement by the sickfund is done on presentation of a certificate of medical care delivered by the practitioner, mentioning the patient's identity and the necessary information for the sickfund.
Those administrative data are usually on a label distributed by the sickfund to its members and to be posted on the form and completed by the practitioner by mentioning the nomenclature's code number and the date of the received medical care.
The nomenclature of medical procedures is a list of all reimbursed diagnostic and therapeutic procedures.
It is a 6 digit number and since April 1985 there is a distinct number for both ambulatory and hospital care procedures.

Each code number is attributed a key letter (B.K.N.C...) and a relative value e.g. E.C.G.=475075 (ambulatory) and 475086 (hospital patient) = K 25(K = 22,2802bf). The reimbursement is 557 BF- E.C.G. being a procedure on the list of major risks and reimbursed at 100%. Restrictions are embedded in the nomenclature prescriptions in order to prevent abuses. The major cause of abuses however is the third party payer where the patient has no direct control. It is widely believed that immediate payment by the patient to his doctor could save quite some money but this measure is vehemently opposed by the sickfunds and the workers unions. Only for hospitalized patients a copy of the invoice has to be handed over to the patient.

Other restrictions are concerned with reservation of certain procedures for a given medical discipline.
E.C.G. is reimbursed for all internists and cardiologists but only to those G.P.s who have acquired an additional license for electrocardiography.
All patients can claim reimbursement for all medical procedures if the physician is accredited with the Ministry of Social Affairs.
The doctor has to be registered with the "Provinciale Raad van de Orde der Geneesheren" and with the "Provinciale Geneeskundige Commissie", which is the provincial branch of the Ministry of Health. This medical committee issues a licence to the doctor to practice medicine in its territory when he supplies an authorized copy of his diploma. With the licence and his diploma he will obtain an inscription in the list of the Provinciale Raad van de Orde and then he is able to settle down and open a medical practice wherever he chooses to do so.
For the reimbursement of his patients he goes to the R.I.Z.I.V. (National Institute for Health and Disability Insurance) where he will be receiving a booklet containing the certificates of medical care he has to issue to his patients. Specialists need besides the above mentioned attributes the accreditation from the board of their medical speciality.

The fees for hospital care are increasingly paid by the sickfunds directly to the practitioners (third party payer). In the majority of hospitals management organizes the billing for the doctors to the sickfunds. In most hospitals the newcoming specialist has to give up his right of collecting himself the fees with his patients. Hospital management is allowed to charge 6 % for this "service" whereas service bureaus offer the same service at 1,5 % or 2 %.
On the other hand most hospitals pay the fees to the doctors with considerable delay.

There have been a few scandals lately. The sickfunds receive the money to pay for doctors' services and hospital costs from the R.I.Z.I.V. With good documented charges the leader of the major doctors union proved that some of the sickfunds delayed the payment of the received sums in order to gain handsome interests from the banks. The hospitals - as well as many doctors - are desperately short of cash and have to lend the money from their bank. The profits accumulated by the sickfunds are said to reach several hundreds of millions of Belgian francs.
Sofar the Minister of Social Affairs has declared that the disputed procedure can be appreciated as "good management" since sickfunds explained that it was only during weekends that they put the money in the bank.

Critics charge that hospitals have to pay interest during weekends too and that it should not take more time to transfer the money to its owners (hospital, doctors) as to transfer it to a very lucrative account in their bank. Another charge is that more than 4 billion Belgian francs have been spend for which the sickfunds could not give a satisfying explanation. Sofar there is no verdict, the investigations continue.

7. Medical documentation

The Code of Medical Ethics prescribes the obligation of keeping a medical record for each patient, but it says nothing about its form and very little about its contents.

Information on drugs is given by the Ministry of Health. Medical registration (The Minimum Medical Record) is mandatory for university hospitals but several hospitals outside the university cooperate to this on a voluntary basis.
There are only limited results for the hospitals involved.

8. Governmental and non-governmental organizations and professional bodies

We have a Ministry of Social Affairs which includes the former Ministry of Public Health (now state secretariat) and the Ministry of Social Security.
The Ministry supervises the R.I.Z.I.V. - the National Institute for Health and Disability Insurance.
Under the R.I.Z.I.V. umbrella are the sickfunds which are for their majority linked with the political parties and their workers unions.
The Christian sickfunds cover +/- 45 % of the population.
The Socialist :+/- 25 %.
The Liberals :+/- 6 %
Professionals :+/- 12 %
Neutrals :+/- 9 %
Auxiliary fund: < 1 %
Railroad :+/- 2 %

The premiums for health-care insurance are paid by the employers directly to the National Insurance Institute.The government adds to that sum an ever decreasing sum coming from taxes (e.g. on tobacco). The National Institute pays the sickfunds and those pass the reimbursements to the patients almost immediately upon presentation of the certificate for given care which has been handed to them by their doctor. Payment to hospitals and to physicians for hospitalized patient care, is done with considerable delay which can exceed 6 months.
The Ministry of Public Health has national and regional branches.

Professional bodies

Several scientific organizations for G.P.s and for the different specialities exist.
There are also unions for all doctors as well as for G.P.s and specialists.
Almost all organizations are regionalised(Flemish-Frenchspeaking).
Our Medical Informatics Association (MIM) is still a national one.

Computers:

Computer usage in the doctor's office is still limited - less than 1%. This may be a surprise to some people who surely remember papers by our colleague Dr. G. Temmerman on early applications for aid in diagnosis and preventive medicine for general practitioners. Among the reasons there is at first the continuously deteriorating financial situation of the medical profession. In other countries it seems that a major argument for selling office computers to physicians is the improvement of the financial administration of the doctor's practice which by itself justifies the investment.
In Belgium the patient pays his doctor in the office and there is no need for sophisticated electronic equipment for recording or follow-up for that purpose.

Specialists who have a lot of reporting to do can use a computer for word-processing and for patient administration.
For family physicians an incentive can be found in the possibility of an improvement in the quality of the care given to their patients for which there is no reward from the sickfunds but which will be appreciated by their patients.
However, a doctor with only a limited number of patients simply cannot afford the investment.

The scientific organizations cannot be blamed for lack of interest since M.I.M (medical informatics) as well as the Flemish- and Frenchspeaking organizations for family physicians organized symposia on medical informatics in general and in particular for computers in the doctor's office.
Both W.V.V.H.(Scientific Organization of Flemish Family Physicians) and S.S.M.G.(Societe Scientifique des Medecins Generalistes) have organized highly successful meetings for their members in 1983.
There was indeed great interest for the new technology but the existing programs did not appeal to the vast majority.
In December 1984 at a joint meeting of the three mentioned organizations the results of an inquiry regarding the use of office computers by the medical profession were communicated.
What follows are the comments on that inquiry's results.

The results concern only a limited sample.
There are only very few applications in our country - less than 1% use a computer in their practice. The coding of the medical activity is of interest to only a small percentage of the physicians.
What is recorded will probably never come out of the doctor's practice.
The preferences expressed by the future users indicate a lack of insight in the possibilities of medical informatics.
Word-processing and access to information networks are most prominent on the future users' list. Another conclusion is that most physicians are waiting for programs that do not require any special effort from a future user.
Only half of the interrogated show an interest for recording the medical record.
Of those claiming to use their computer for the medical record, a majority is using an unstructured record system.
P.O.M.R. (Problem Oriented Medical Record) is used by quite a few G.P.s but is almost unknown to specialists.
The final conclusion was that the scientific organisations M.I.M.-W.V.V.H. and S.S.M.G. still have a lot of work to do in order to promote medical informatics among their membership. But before that both practice analysis and a well structured medical record system are necessary. Otherwise it will be "garbage in, garbage out".

As a conclusion I would say that mainly for cost reasons medical informatics in Belgium has still a very long way to go.
But there is also a need for more user-friendly programs.
There are no restrictions for import from abroad but the very specific situation of the medical profession in Belgium makes it quite difficult for imported programs to succeed.
On the other hand the financial problems are there for the Belgian products as well but besides that an investment for a good program is too heavy a risk for most Belgian companies in view of the relatively small number of possible purchasers.On top of those difficulties comes the fact that our country is further divided by two languages (Flemish- and French- speaking physicians). Nevertheless there are a few programs that are both well structured and user-friendly and that probably will succeed.

A suggestion has been launched lately for a special reimbursement for a quality medical record. This is based on the fact that a special reimbursement already exists for "the written report" from a specialist to a referring general practitioner. This reimbursement of 326 BF for each report resulted in an overnight compliance with the wish of the general practitioners to become both better and faster informed by the consultant specialist.

References
----

1. Blanpain J, Lindgren B, Sandier S (1985)
Comparaisons internationales des systemes de sante. CREDES

2. Inkomensbeleid voor geneesheren (1983)
Mededelingen nr.10 - A.S.G.B. Van Putlei 13 - B-2018 Antwerpen

3. Temmerman G. (1980)
Some automated record models with logical and logistical support for high standard general practice.
The computer in the doctor's office -Eds. O. Rienhoff and M. E. Abrams, North-Holland Publ. Co., Amsterdam

4. L'automatisation du resume de dossier medical en medecine generale. Rapport presente par Dr. E. Degraeve (1982)
Programmatie van het Wetenschapsbeleid
(Wetenschapsstraat 8 - B-1040 BRUSSELS)

5. Automatisatie Medisch Dossier Huisarts
Wetenschappelijk verslag samengesteld door Dr. W. Peumans (1982)
Programmatie wetenschapsbeleid
(Wetenschapsstraat 8 - B-1040 BRUSSELS)

6. Statistisch Jaarboek van Volksgezondheid -dienstjaar 1983
Centrum voor Informatieverwerking
Ministerie van Volksgezondheid en van het Gezin
Rijksadministratief centrum- Vesaliusgebouw, B-1000 BRUSSELS

7. Wijnen A. La paille et la poutre 1982/1985
Bulletin Syndical - rue du Chateau 15, B-1420 Braine-l'Alleud

8. Computergebruik in de ambulante praktijk (1984)
Results of the inquiry by M.I.M.(medical informatics association) presented by W. Peumans
G.Verwilghensingel 4 - B-3500 Hasselt

SYSTEMS IN PRIMARY CARE IN FRANCE

Dr. Francois Dumont, Dr. Pierre Gallois
Unaformec-France, 311, rue Lecourbe, F-75015 Paris

0. INTRODUCTION

In 1981, Dr. Pierre Gallois, Chairman of Unaformec (National Union of Medical Continuous Training Associations), and the main author of this address, opened his major report on the organization of care systems by quoting from the French philosopher and scientist Pascal as follows: "a sphere, the center of which is everywhere, and the circumference nowhere"; this was Dr. Gallois' way of illustrating the French health system.

This system is not easy to describe in a static way. It is made up of a multitude of health care professionals with objectives, statutes and various specializations, who individually generate their own networks of health care, communication, and even financial flow.

Each one of these medical actors can use two, three or four modes of practice, and belong to as many management systems. Approximately half the doctors relate to this study because of their duties as ambulatory doctors, have, in the same way, one or more methods of practice.

Because of the many inconsistencies in the statistics at hand, we have only chosen the most important trends and figures.

Due to the vastness of the subject and the relatively short size of this paper, it was not possible for us to quote our sources at each step.

As a general rule, our concern to present a comprehensive presentation while following the given outline led us to resort to rough estimates or use partial examples when precise data were non-existent; this, of course, while differentiating between the various categories of statistics.

1. THE STRUCTURE OF PRIMARY CARE

1.1 Who delivers primary care, where and when

We call primary care a first resort, due to an initiative taken by the part of the patient or those around him, thus excluding medical care given as a consequence of the request of another doctor.

Arbitrarily we are also excluding primary care given by hospital outpatient services or hospital emergency services which, in spite of their relative importance, (which is, in fact, decreasing) pose different problems from those relating to the objectives of this study.

1.2 Number of physicians in ambulatory primary care

Statistics are difficult to analyze due to the unclear part played by specialists in the field of primary care, and the important percent of part-time hospital practitioners whose outside activities are poorly surveyed, thus including a portion of primary care.

The statistics provided for 1980 by the French medical association (total number of individuals in July 1980) showed that of the 109.070 practicing doctors:

- 46.955 were general practitioners, and
- 50.235 were specialists.

The remainder of professionals were not practitioners in the therapeutic field. Furthermore, 35.065 house physicians were listed at that time, of which:

- 15.797 worked full-time in hospitals, and
- 19.268 worked part-time.

About 1.000 G.P. are full-time salaried doctors in county health centers.

1.2.1 Physicians

Primary care as defined above, is administered by general practitioners, as it is their vocation, almost exclusively. 66 % of primary care is administered in their private consultation offices, and 34 % of cases on calls at the patient's home.

Office consultations and house calls stretch from about 8 am to 8 pm. Practitioners remain on call at night and on Sundays and holidays. This service is usually organized on a rotation basis among the practitioners of a given area, or provided by autonomous call and emergency organizations.

Specialists, (this does not include specialists who practice in public hospitals) very often work on a first resort basis. Statistics vary according to the individual, the specialty and the region, therefore it is difficult to provide figures. However, it seems that taken as a whole only 15% of a specialist's practice results from the request of a general practitioner (this fact does not rule out the setting up of an agreement between the specialist and the general practitioner for a portion of the 85 % of consultations carried out by direct access).

In the vast majority of cases, specialists treat their patients in their offices. House calls made by specialists only represent 1,5 % of all specialized medical treatment (and 2 % of the general total of house calls, as the remaining 98 % are still carried out by general practitioners).

Specialists receive patients in their offices generally on the basis of pre-scheduled appointments. Services providing specialized care for emergency duty at night and on Sundays and holidays are of the second resort type, in other words without direct access from the part of the public (excluding public or private hospitals).

Full-time house physicians not being included in the scope of our study, the number of specialists practicing medicine on a first resort basis can be estimated at about 35.000.

The percentage of practitioners contributing to primary care can be estimated as follows:

57% are general practitioners,
43% are specialists.

But even if the activity of general practitioners rests almost exclusively on primary care, it is very difficult, as we have already seen, to define the share of a specialist's activity taken up by primary care.

We have estimated this share at 84 % of their consultation and at 33 % of first resort medical treatment. (These figures were computed from data provided by the National Health Insurance Fund relative to the total of medical consultations carried out by general practitioners and medical specialists in 1983.)

1.2.2 Participation of allied health personnel

Medical secretaries.
We were not able to find statistics on the number of medical secretaries. It seems that each group practice employs one or more secretaries (there are 8.500 group practices). In single-doctor practices a secretary is employed but on a less constant basis.

Nurses.
(Source: National health insurance fund 1983). In the majority of cases, nurses work on an independent basis even if they are based in a group practice. There are 24.021 independent nurses. Furthermore, surveys show that there are 1.284 nursing care clinics employing salaried nurses. In addition, there are 403 health care centers employing nurses.

Physiotherapists.
(Source: National health insurance fund 1983). There are 22.848 physiotherapists practicing on a free-lance basis, in private offices for the most part. Only 114 practice in "societe civile" or professional partnerships.

Other independent medical auxiliaries.

speech therapists 4.639,
orthopedists 741.

2. CATCHMENT AREAS AND ACCESS FOR PATIENTS

Health care is allocated in France on the general principle that the patient is free to choose his or her doctor.
There is therefore no geographical sectoring imposed on the public. The only restriction applicable to this freedom of choice on the part of patients lies in the reimbursement conditions concerning doctor's fees for travelling to and from house calls, as the patient is reimbursed according to the distance between his or her home and the closest practitioner.

In the field of psychiatric care given by doctors in the public sector, a system of districts exists. By law it is not imposed on patients but in practice it is difficult for patients to be treated beyond the bounds of their district.

3. STRUCTURES OF PRACTICES

A survey carried out by the French national council of the medical association in 1979 showed that on a total of 68.395 independent doctors,

58 % worked alone,
36 % practiced in group offices,
6 % worked on an exclusive basis in private clinics.

4. PRINCIPLES OF REMUNERATION

As regards primary care, the system is based on the patient paying the practitioner directly and at the time of the consultation.

In some cases the practitioner is paid by a third party, in this case by the health insurance fund and not by the patient. This applies to labor accidents, persons benefiting from public assistance, and free health care for war victims. This system of payment through a third party is also applicable to major forms of treatment (surgery, radiology) or certain prescriptions for drugs or tests, depending on agreements between professional organizations and insurance health funds.

Finally, in particular health care schemes, such as those applicable in the mining or railway professions, the practitioners are salaried and treat patients chosen on lists (for mining funds) or employed in their district (for railway funds). However, patients can seek treatment with another doctor and be refunded in most cases.

5. STRUCTURE OF PATIENTS

5.1 Insurance status

Almost all the French are affiliated with the social health insurance program. This social security system is based upon the reimbursement of medical and pharmaceutical treatment at a rate of 70 %. In the event of hospitalization exceeding 30 days, patients can be refunded at a rate of 100 %, as well as in some cases on important intervention such as surgical operations, including appendicitis.

Furthermore, 100 % reimbursement of all health care is possible for a certain number of long-term illnesses (this form of refund is specified by a list of 26 illnesses), and in the case of particulary costly care, patients can receive 100 % refunds for labor accidents or occupational diseases.

Aside from the standard social security system, there are special systems for railway workers, servicemen, miners, agricultural laborers, or non-salaried or non-agricultural workers, whose rates and methods of reimbursement vary from one system to another.

Finally, supplementary insurance systems are available to individuals or certain professions; mutual insurance or private insurance systems thus ensure that the portion of fees which is not reimbursed by social health is refunded to the member, and in particular the 30% refunded for primary care.

Special systems are set up for the needy or for wounded war veterans.

5.2 Morbidity spectrum

A survey carried out by CREDOC on therapeutic morbidity in ambulatory medicine on 1.400 general practitioners and specialists in 1980 provided the following information:

(1) 11,5 % of treatment is preventive, in the broad sense of the term, and includes 2,3 % for systematic consultations for newborns, 2,2 % for contraception, 1,8 % for vaccinations, 1,7 % for administrative reasons, etc..

(2) One out of two medical consultations is due to a single reason, close to 8 % are due to 4 reasons or more.

(3) 58 % of patients seeking medical care are women, 42 % men. Female doctors have more female patients (65 %) than male doctors (57 %).
Elderly people over 65 make up 19 % of patients, but are 25,6 % of a general practitioner's clientele.

(4) Reasons for seeking medical attention from a general practitioner are as follows:

- cardiovascular diseases 37,4 % (including hypertension 12,3 %)
- mental disorders and insomnia 18,5 % (including 4,9 % for insomnia)
- locomotor apparatus 18,4 %
- digestive tract 16,4 %
- general symptoms 16,2 % (including asthenia 4,2 %)
- ear, nose, throat 15,4 %
- prevention 13,6 %
- endocrinic-diabetic 8,9 %
- respiratory system 8,4 %
- traumatism 7,2 %
- genital-urinary diseases 6,9 %
- dermatology 5,3 %
- infectious diseases 4,8 %
- tumours 3,3 %
- pregnancy 1,8 %
- miscellaneous 4,2 %.

(5) In 76 % of cases medication is prescribed, containing an average of 2,8 different drugs.
The same survey carried out in July 1983 showed that 3,3 drugs were prescribed. In both cases the method for computing this statistic is not given; it is not known whether this figure applies to medication, the cost of which is refunded by social security at either 100 % or 70 %, so-called "comfort" drugs with a lesser rate of reimbursement, or renewals of long-term prescriptions. General practitioners in several regions have taken

the initiative of carrying out more in-depth surveys on the question.

(6) In 14,9 % of cases biological tests are prescribed, X-rays in 5,5 % of cases, and in 5,9 % of cases consultation with another doctor is recommended.

(7) A survey carried out by INSERM in 1975 showed the following distribution of reasons for consulting a general practitioner:

- acute diseases 25 %
- chronic diseases 40 %
- functional disorders 25 %
- prevention-administrative 10 %.

The majority of patients with chronic illnesses are elderly. Distribution is as follows:

- hypertension 10 %
- diabetes 4,5 %
- bronchitis 2,6 %
- cerebrovascular 2,5 %
- etc..

6. MANDATORY DOCUMENTATION FOR ACCOUNTING

There is a nomenclature of medical treatment used to bill medical care. Each procedure has a code, as follows:

- C for consulting a doctor in his office
  (C = general practitioner
  CS = specialist
  Cpsy = psychiatrist)
- V for house calls (also includes VS and Vpsy)
- K for diagnostic or therapeutic treatment. This code varies according to the nature of the treatment as follows:
  K5 = plural puncture
  K6.5 = electrocardiogram
  K50 = appendectomy
- Z for X-rays, the code varying according to the type of treatment.
- B for biological tests, the code varying according to the type of treatment.

Furthermore, treatment in the K category is preceded by another code depending on the speciality (for example, CHI for surgery).

Each key letter (C.V.K.Z.B.) corresponds to a rate which is determined following an agreement between unions representing doctors and social security funds (governmental approval is, however, necessary).

The practitioner's travelling expenses for house calls are reimbursed according to a series of coefficients, taking into account the size of the town, the distance covered and the nature of the therapy.

Practitioners have the right to exceed conventional rates in a certain number of cases:

- A particular requirement on the part of the patient. The code DE must then be added onto the health insurance form.

- "Notoriety" as recognized by official bodies. The code is DP as this signifies a "droit permanent", or permanent right, to charge more than conventional fees. This right was abolished in the last convention arrived at between doctors and social security bodies, however, those who had acquired this right in the past are still allowed to enforce it.

- The choice of "secteur II" stipulated in the most recent agreement. In this case, the practitioner is free to determine his fees "with tact and moderation". Patients are reimbursed following conventional rates; however, they do not benefit from certain social advantages.

- Non-conventionalization. The patient is reimbursed for prescription expenses, but not for medical treatment.

  12,8 % of general practitioners belong to the last 3 categories, 1,2 % of which are non-conventionalized.

There are no clauses restricting the social security system's taking patients in charge. However, the following should be pointed out:

- If free care is administered to a patient because he is a war victim, the case will not be taken in charge by the social security system.

- Travelling costs occurring when a doctor makes a house call are reimbursed following the distance between the patient's home and the nearest doctor.

However, private insurance schemes involve exclusion clauses formulated at the time the contract is signed concerning certain illnesses, or the date the illness began in relation to the signature of the contract.

7. MANDATORY LEGAL DOCUMENTATION

No person can claim to be a medical practitioner if he or she is not listed on the Ordre des Medecins, or French medical association, chart. This, however, does not apply to doctors working as civil servants who have no private patients.

All doctors with private patients must be members of the Caisse Autonome de Retraite des Medecins Francais, or autonomous French doctors' retirement fund: Membership fees are calculated according to a complex rate system which is far too detailed to be listed here.

Last of all, a certain number of regulations control the settlement of young doctors. It is also mandatory for medical doctors' diplomas to be registered with administrative authorities.

- There are no recertification or specific quality requirements.

- There are no legal requirements for medical records, but a medical record must exist.

8. STATUS OF COMPUTER SUPPORT IN THE COUNTRY

There are three basic systems applying data processing in France:

- remote message processing, or telematics,
- individual microcomputing,
- microcomputing coupled with remote message processing.

8.1
Remote message processing or "telematics" is the answer to the public authorities wish to develop electronic communication by telephone on the public packet network (which also enables written data to be exchanged using a keyboard and a visual display unit linked to any telephone line).

This implies:

- Resorting to large computers ("servers" or information retrieval systems) capable of managing a data bank as well as the essential communication procedures.

- Standardization of transmission and equipment norms on the market.

In the field of health care, the first data banks were scientific, and used by research centers. In the past two years, however, new products geared towards the general medical public have appeared for use by doctors not practising in the hospital sector (approximately 80.000).

Trade publications, such as the Quotidien du Medecin, have had a telematic journal available since 1984, as well as an electronic mail service. Cadutique, a publication specialized in health care data processing, has on offer a medical information service (congresses, message transmission via the Cadutel network available to subscribers, etc...). Other firms like Meditex, or the Serveur Medical, offer similar services and are trying to group electronic mailing services to make them available to typical professional bodies such as the French medical association, or the unions.

Access to these services is expensive, but the cost is in fact much lower than the actual cost (approximately 10 %). This implies resorting to financial backing from the pharmaceutical industry, or public subsidies. This logical situation is presently going through a "breaking-in" phase, and will probably not continue as such. One can rightfully wonder how users will react once they will have to actually pay for the service (at a cost of approximately 300 Francs per month per user).

In Sept. 1985, 30 medical servers or data banks using Videotex transmission have been listed, at different costs.

Electronic mail services can thus organize descriptive epidemiology surveys for a particular region pertaining to the server. Furthermore, this type of terminal enables doctors to have access to all the other data banks such as the Biam (or automated computerized drug data bank). This vast therapeutic file is continuously updated, and was launched on an experimental basis in 1984 by 150 doctors in the Bordeaux region.

This is extending because terminals "Minitel" are lent free of charge by French telecommunication services to many professions including doctors.

8.2
Personal microcomputing is typical of those pioneers whose wish it was to computerize the management of their office information systems, in other words medical file management, accounting, word processing or appointment scheduling. These data processing systems developed in a totally anarchistic way. Efforts on the part of the medical profession did not go beyond the dispatching of a brochure to 50.000 doctors working outside the hospital sector, in order to make them aware of the situation. This followed a trade gathering called the Clim, or liaison committee for computerized medical information, which brought together the French medical association, the medical unions, Unaformec and medical data processing clubs.

It is impossible to evaluate how many doctors have microcomputers. However, through medical file management software package sales, it is known that 1.500 doctors have purchased these packages, approximately twenty of which are presently marketed. Four of these packages share 3/4 of the market on a very irregular basis, and the investment varies between 25.000 to 85.000 francs. However, one must point out that the latest studies taken among the medical profession show that, due to the increasing impoverishment (more doctors and poorly assessed fees) of practitioners, it is no longer possible to invest such large amounts. This trend is going to radically change development perspectives for data processing in the field of ambulatory medicine in the coming years.

Actually, penetration of microcomputers among practitioners is about 2 %.

8.3
The third system available to doctors is that of lower-end microcomputing, either configurated or via a telematic terminal. This system functions either by teleloading information or by sharing certain data with other confreres; this is possible if they own compatible equipment (the Apple medical club has 450 users).

9. CONCLUSION

All things considered, a certain consistency of opinion vis a vis the positive aspects of the data processing tool, particularly in the field of data communication, seems to be taking shape. However, the widespread use of data processing systems is hindered by cultural as well as financial problems. French doctors are by nature individualistic, and neither like sharing medical data nor having to question their work habits.

The purpose of continuous medical education associations (Unaformec) in medical informatics is to find computerized services giving response to the needs in office practice.

System analysis of primary care in Italy: perspectives and problems of computerized information systems

F. de Rosis

Health Information Systems, Istituto di Scienze dell' Informazione, Università, Via Amendola 173
Bari, Italy

INTRODUCTION

The National Health Service creation Act of 1978 has defined common criteria of access to health care of the whole population, in the spirit of an egalitarian principle of 'health safeguard as a right of the individual and as an interest of the collectivity', which has to be guaranteed by the State to all its citizens.

According to this Act, the enrollment in the NHS is compulsory to everybody: however, private insurances are also allowed. The National Health Service is organized in various levels of decentralization (National, Regional, Local): the USL (Unità Sanitaria Locale, Local Health Unit) is responsible for the health care of a population ranging from 20.000 to 250.000 inhabitants (80.000 on the average). In particular, it takes care of administrative relationships with the population and the health personnel.

The Act acknowledges the central role of prevention and primary health care. Some of these functions are covered by NHS employees working in ad hoc services (e.g. environmental hygiene, work environment health and safety, maternal and child welfare, vaccinations, care of the elderlies and the handicapped). But the predominant part of this sector lies in the responsibility for a network of general practitioners who are linked to the Service by a triennial Contract: i.e., the doctors who have the required titles may be inscribed in regional pass-lists and are assigned to a specific USL. At the moment of the enrollment into the NHS, every member of the population has to choose one of the g.p.s being in the list of his USL of residence (or, exceptionally, of another USL); this choice is generally extended to the other family members: therefore, the g.p. is usually a 'family doctor'.

General practitioners are responsible for the individual preventive medicine, health care and education of their patients, in the respect of guidelines issued from the National or the Regional Health Plans. This activity is not compatible with an employment of more than 38 hours per week, nor with an activity as full-time specialist: however, these regulations do not limit the possibility, for a doctor, to have private patients.

The general practitioner receives a remuneration per capita, based on the number of patients who have chosen him. The last Contract establishes a maximum number of patients that every doctor is allowed to take on: 1500 for a doctor who has no other activity (which can be raised up to 1800 in particular cases), 500 for those who have a part-time employment.

This number is inversely proportional (for all other cases) to the number of hours spent in other employments.

The general practitioner has, among his duties, the role of regulating the partially free of charge supply of other health services: in particular, the supply of drugs by the pharmacy and the access to most specialist diagnostic or therapeutic facilities is conditioned to a 'prescription' by a g.p. enrolled with the National Health Service.

1. STRUCTURE OF PRIMARY CARE

A study made in 1984 by Splendori shows that Italy has a great number of doctors (220.000 for a population of 57 millions inhabitants): this number has progressively grown in the last 10 years, whereas the population was relatively stable; in the same years, the number of students who entered the Faculty of Medicine has decreased regularly, also as a result of an information campaign of the professional organizations, which signalized the risks of a massive unemployment in this sector (see Fig. 1).

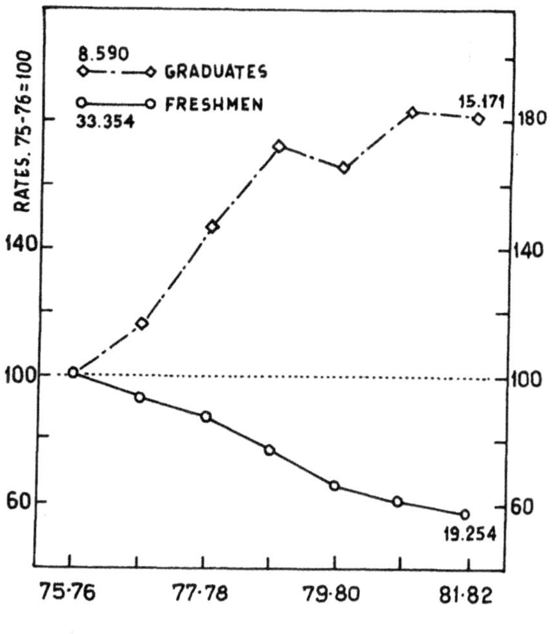

Fig. 1. No. of students who obtained a degree in medicine from 75 to 82 and no. of students who entered the faculty, in the same period. Source: Splendori 1984.

The age distribution of doctors is given in Fig. 2: it shows a nearly bimodal distribution, with a higher first peak centered on the class 30-31: 60 % of doctors are below 40 years of age.

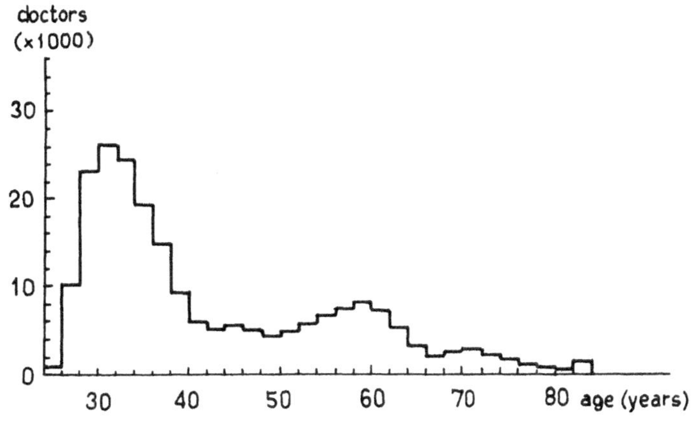

Fig. 2. Age distribution of doctors in 1984. Source: Splendori 1984

Nearly the same percentage of doctors work as general practitioners (73.000 : 33 %) and in hospitals or universities (89.000 : 41 % ; see Table 1). Following an estimate from the FIMG (Federation of General Practitioners, see paragraph 8), there are about 50.000 young doctors who have not still reached the titles which are needed to enter the lists of the National Health Service, and who are totally or partially unemployed.

Table 1. No. of doctors by their prevalent activity. Source: Splendori 1984.

type of activity	doctors x 1000
public employees	
university	11
hospitals	78
public health	11
under contract with the NHS	
general practitioners	73
specialists	30
private employees	unknown

The doctors-to-inhabitants ratio is favourable to the patients (the highest in the European Communities, see Fig. 3). This ratio is also high for primary care: about 900 inhabitants per g.p. (Ministero della Sanità 1985). However, the distribution of patients among the g.p.s is extremely inhomogeneous: the southern and central regions have a higher proportion of doctors than the nord and the islands. In addition (see Fig. 4), there is a percentage of g.p.s who have a great number of patients (still greater than the maximum allowed), at the expenses of an 'army' of young doctors who are only officially in the market (having very few patients in their lists).

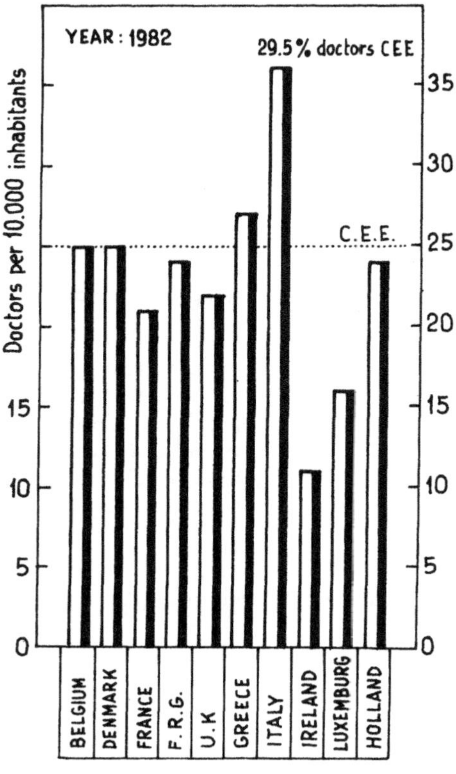

Fig. 3. No. of doctors per 10 thousand inhabitants in the European Communities.
Source: Splendori 1984.

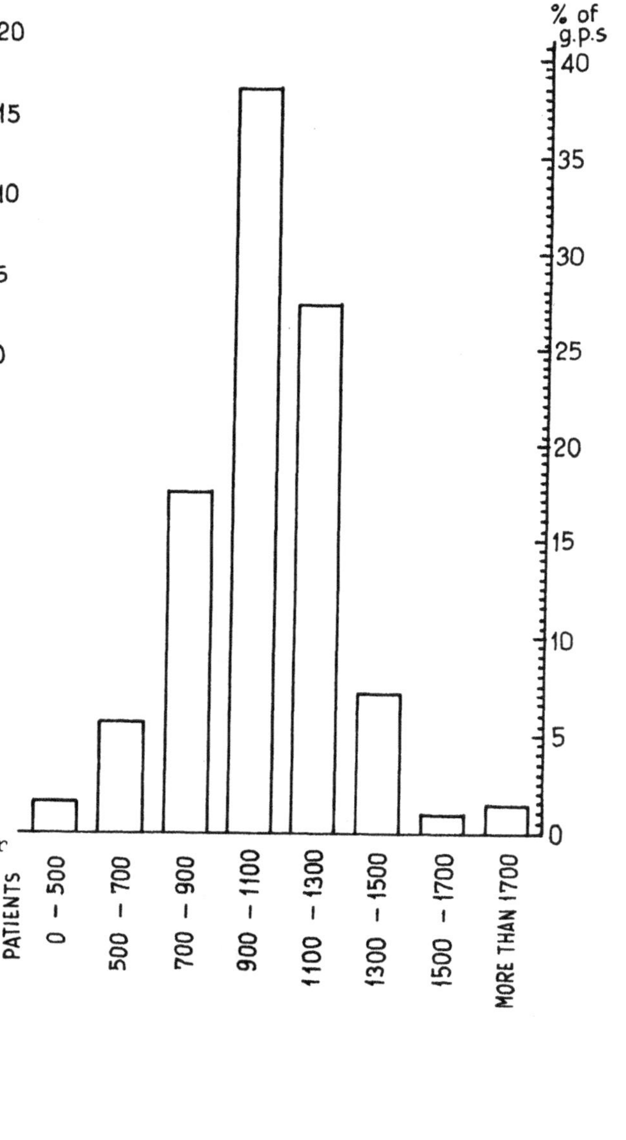

Fig.4. Distribution of g.p.s under contract with the NHS, by the number of patients in their lists.
Source: Ministero della Sanità 1985.

This situation is more serious in large cities: following an inquiry of 1980, which covered all the 5000 g.p.s of Rome (de Rosis 1984), a 12 % of g.p.s (having more than 1500 patients) withholded a 42 % of the population, in an evident situation of 'monopole', whereas about 31 % had less than 50 patients and 14 % had no patients at all: the number of patients was significantly related to the age of the doctor (see Fig. 5). A more uniform distribution of patients among the doctors has been reached in these years, as a result of the limitation of the maximum number of patients which was fixed by the Contract.

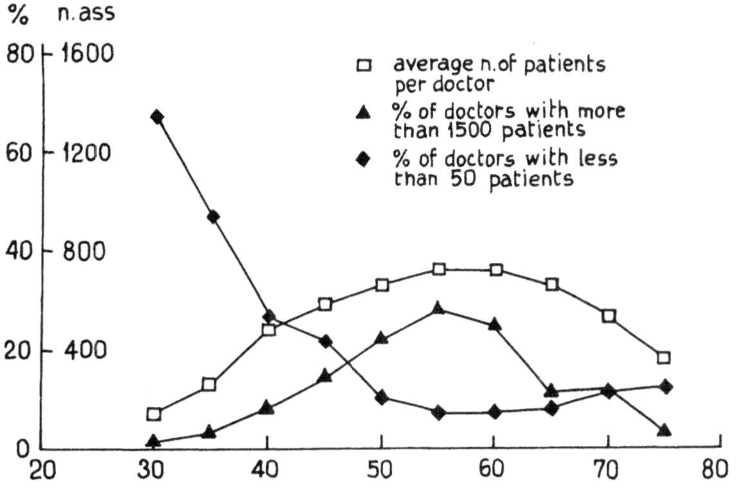

Fig. 5. Relationship between number of patients in the list and doctor's age (city of Rome, 1980). Source : de Rosis 1984.

A survey of 1980 by the Department of Health (which covered 49 % of g.p.s in Italy) shows that 47 % of them had another employment (and therefore a reduced maximum of patients allowed: Ministero della Sanità 1984). The proportion of doctors who practice as g.p.s though having a specialization is not known.

The personnel working in the ambulatory is linked to the doctor by a private contract. Their medical qualification is generally poor (this is a major problem also in the public health sector in Italy); when the doctor has more than 800-900 patients, he generally employs a nurse with secretarial or cleaning duties; very unfrequently, however, he entrusts her with medical responsibilities.

The total health expenditure in 1984 was of about 37.000 billions of lire (360 dollars per inhabitant):the primary care covers only 7 % of this figure.

2. STRUCTURE OF THE POPULATION

The distribution of the population in the three age classes which are relevant to the activity and to the remuneration of the g.p.s is as follows: 15 % under 12, 19 % over 60, 66 % adults. The age pyramids in southern and northern regions are much different (see Fig. 6), the southern regions having a higher rate of birth.

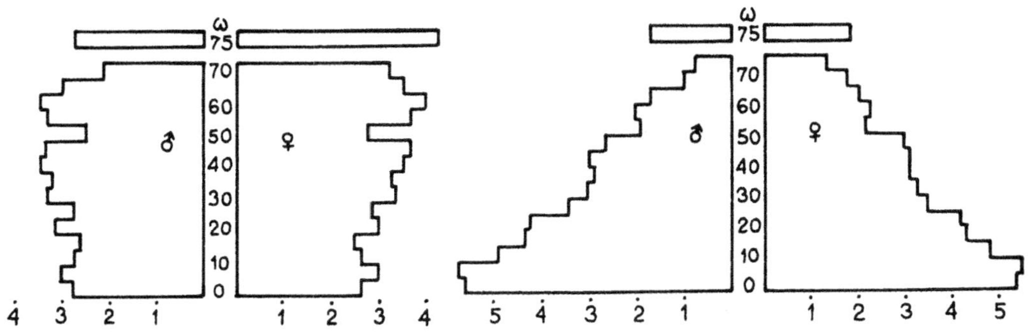

Fig. 6. Age pyramids in a northern (leftside) and a southern (rightside) region.

The National Institute of Statistics (ISTAT) gives regular information only on the mortality of the population: detailed morbidity statistics are not available, with the exception of infectious diseases subject to compulsory notification.

Death rates show that serious territorial and social inequalities in the risk of death still exist in Italy: northern regions are in a situation typical of industrialized countries (prevalence of chronic and degenerative diseases), whereas the rate of infant mortality and the incidence of some infectious diseases in southern regions is still at levels of developing countries : see Fig.7 (Berlinguer 1983).

The citizen chooses his general practitioner at the USL's administrative bureau. He can change this choice in every moment, although this does not seem to happen very frequently: according to the evaluation of the FIMG, changes are especially due to transfers of residence, and therefore are more frequent in large cities; not more than 10 % of patients seem to change their g.p. in a year, on the average.

3. STRUCTURE OF PRACTICES

Doctors have usually a single practice: some of them have more than one practice, in different USLs. No official figures are available on the frequency of mixed professional practices, but this type of work seems to be unfrequent.

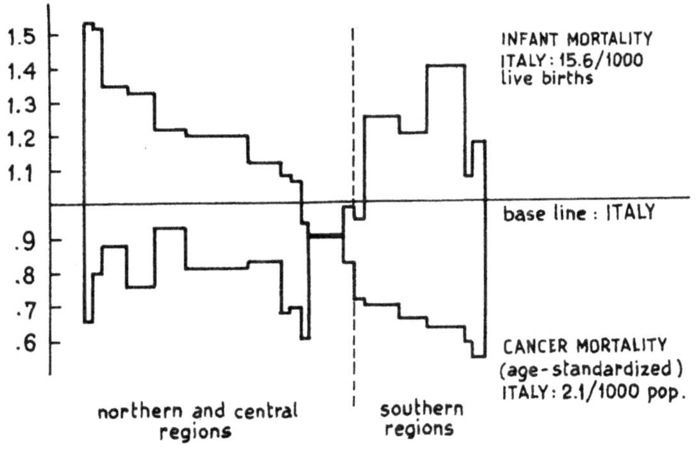

Fig. 7. Ratios of regional vs national death rates for two conditions. Source: Annuario Statistico ISTAT 1980, re-elaboration.

Following the first Projects of National Health Plans (formulated shortly after the National Health Service creation Act), services similar to the English Health Centers had to be organized in the District (the most peripheral node of the NHS, which should cover a population of about 10.000 inhabitants): however, this objective has always been postponed, and, so far, there has been no public initiative aimed at favouring an integration of the activity of g.p.s with that of public services engaged in primary care.

The obligation, which was introduced by the first Contract, to respect a maximum number of patients frequently not corresponding to the actual situation, has forced the doctors who were out of the rules to associate to their practice one or more young doctors, in order to entrust them with a part of their patients. The Contract mentions that a maximum of 4 general practitioners and 1 pediatrician could associate, and that the USL should establish non economical incentives of cooperation among associated doctors, in initiatives concerning training, health education and research. The number of practices with associated doctors is high (about 5000). However, usually the association has not implied a different style of work, and has been considered only as a temporary expedient to come into the Law without loosing the confidence of the patients: with the time, associated doctors should all acquire these patients in their lists, and should assume an independent status.

The possibility to organize group practices is also mentioned in the Contract, with the objective of 'improving the quality of care and of insuring a coordinated and more effective fulfillment of activities'. The exact terms of this practice, however, have never been defined. Therefore, initiatives of this type are still rare: two seminars have been organized in 1985 by a group of doctors who are very active in this field. The few (but apparently most promising) experiences discussed concerned young doctors who practice in northern Italy: among the objectives which are considered to be of primary importance, there is the possibility to promote a higher qualification of health care, also through a permanent and collective training and auditing, and a common epidemiological work. The perspective to reduce the expenses using common structures and means and to rationalize the work by a suitable subdivision of duties are non secondary incentives: the organisation of a common file of medical records is considered as an indispensable tool to these aims.

To evaluate whether there is a real possibility to extend these experiences out of the limited circles where they have grown until now, it should be mentioned that an inquiry among 1500 general practitioners revealed that, in spite of the lack of any initiative of information and sustain of this style of work, 41 % of interviewed declared to be in favour of the group practice; this percentage was lower in the age group over 50 years of age (30 %) and for those who had more than 1500 patients (33 %; see Panti 1985).

4. REMUNERATION

The capitation fee depends on:

- the doctor's number of postgraduate years (four classes: 0-5; 6-12; 13-20; more than 20);
- the patient's age (three classes: 0-12; 13-60; more than 60).

It also includes an allowance for practice expenses, which covers items like: ambulatory rent, telephone, nurse salary, transportation and 'any other mean which is required to the patient's care'; this contribution corresponds to about 20 % of the total fee, on the average, and is based only on the doctor's declaration (a list of expenditures made, which has to be supported by a copy of the income declaration).

An extra remuneration is due by the Contract, for a number of items of services which are not included among the normal duties of the general practitioner. These activities are listed in the Contract itself: medications, small surgical interventions, treatment of fractures etc; some of them may be required by the USL in substitution of functions that should be covered by its primary care services: e.g. vaccinations and periodical control of workers.

The average monthly remuneration of a doctor who has a Contract as g.p. was, in 1984, of 2.9 millions of lire (about 1600 dollars: Ministero della Sanità 1985): this remuneration corresponds to an average capitation fee of less than two dollars a month. One should remember that this average remuneration resumes an inhomogeneous situation, considering that most of young g.p.s have very few patients, and that this is a second work for many public or private employees.

The Contract establishes that Regional Committees have to be created, with an equal representative of the NHS and of the doctor's organisations, to define the standards of health care that have to be followed and the procedures to verify the quality of care . A Discipline Committee is called to judge those cases where the Contract has been disregarded.

5. STRUCTURE OF PATIENTS

At present, the large majority of inhabitants have chosen their g.p.. The number of private insurance policies is growing, as well as the recourse, on payment, to private services[1], also because of the difficulties in the functioning of the NHS, after the crisis of the Welfare State. However, doctors are consulted privately primarily for a specialist advice, and private policies usually cover only specialist and hospital care. Therefore, one can assume that, today, every citizen has his g.p. and that those g.p.s who take on private work do it as specialists (at least if one considers the activity of primary care in its global sense, and not only for its technical aspects concerning internal medicine).

As we have mentioned in paragraph 2, the knowledge about the morbidity spectrum of the population is not very good in Italy. Two years ago, the ISTAT has organized a special survey on the population's health status (ISTAT 1984) which covered about 31.000 families (a stratified sample of 1.6 % of the population): the results of this survey show that 19.4 % of the interviewed declared to be in a 'not good health status' at the moment of the interview; the interviewed indicated the illnesses shown in Table 2 as responsible of this ill health status.

Table 2. Illnesses and diseases declared by those who are in a 'not good health status' at the moment of the interview (month of November).

diseases and illnesses			%
infectious and parasitic diseases			2.2
psychic troubles			2.8
diseases of the:	nervous	system	2.9
	circulatory	"	7.5
	respiratory	"	40.2
	digestive	"	7.9
	genito-urinary	"	2.6
	musculo-skeletal	"	11.7
ill-defined condition			11.9
accidents-poisoning			3.1
other			3.9
unspecified			3.3

The period chosen for interview does not allow to analyze the importance of chronic diseases with respect to acute diseases.

The same survey showed that the average number of contacts with a g.p. per 100 interviewed, in the first four weeks of the month of November, was equal to 49.7 (see the age and sex distribution in Table 3). Most of these contacts occurred in the practice (65.6 %), but a considerable percentage of them was at domicile (25 %: see Table 4).

1 Following an inquiry of 1984 (Piperno 1986), 46 % of interviewed declared that they used 'sometimes or frequently' private services.

Table 3. Number of contacts with a doctor (per 100 interviewed) in the first 4 weeks of November 1983. Source: ISTAT 1984.

age	0-13	14-49	50-64	over 65	Total
no. of contacts	38	35.5	66.2	95.6	47.9 → 45.6 males; → 53.6 females

Table 4. Types of contacts with a doctor. Source : ISTAT 1984.

type of intervention	% of contacts
domiciliary visit	25.0
ambulatory visit	65.6
telephone contact	2.2
other	1.5
unspecified	5.6

The prevalent reason for these contacts was a disease or illness (60.5 %): control of health status in absence of illness determined 22.2 % of them, whereas it should be mentioned that in 4.7 % of cases a certification or a prescription was the only one reason for the visit (see Table 5). A doctor gives 7 prescriptions of drugs per patient each year, on the average (Ministero della Sanità 1985): but the majority of contacts and prescriptions concern a small section of the population (the aged and the chronic patients who receive drugs free of charge).

Table 5. Reasons that determined a contact with a doctor. Source: ISTAT 1984.

reasons	% of contacts
disease or illness	60.5
control of health status	22.2
certification or other administrative duty	4.7
other	2.5
unspecified	10.1

As a comment to these data, one should mention that the particular period of the year covered in the interview does not allow to make any inference about annual rates: in addition, the inquiry concerned consultations with a doctor, regardless of his specialization: in fact, only 65 % of these consultations was with a general practitioner (the remaining 35 % being with a specialist). Should the rate of contacts be constant during all the year and equal for g.p.s and specialists (which is unlikely), every inhabitant would have about 4 contacts with a g.p. every year (this rate would increase from 3 in the age class 0-12 to 7 in the class over 65).

To integrate this information, one has to use the results of special surveys which have been made on restricted population samples in various regions. Unfortunately, the approaches used are not homogeneous, and therefore the results are not directly comparable. However, they may be used to have an overall picture of the situation, taken from different viewpoints.

An inquiry made in 1979 in the region of Puglia (the boot's heel: Piperno 1981) examined 11.500 consultations made by 200 g.p.s in the months of May and June; it showed: that an equal number of acute (49.8 %) and chronic (45.6 %) problems had been considered in these consultations; that the majority of symptoms presented was considered as 'minor' (67%) or 'negligible' (10 %) by the doctor; that the average duration of a consultation was of 10' in the practice and 22' at domicile (this duration does not seem to be different when the doctor has a second work, which happens for 57 % of them). Only in 4.5 % of cases, a consultation ended without any prescription: in 77.5 % of them, a drug was prescribed, in 2 % a hospital admission, in 9.5 % a laboratory analysis, in 5 % an X-ray. Younger doctors required a specialist's advice more frequently than their older colleagues. It is also noteworthy that, in 32 % of cases, clinical data were registered on a personal record, and that those who had this habit seemed to require with a lower frequency a specialist's diagnostic advice.

Subsequently, in a national stratified sample of 600 inhabitants aged more than 18 years living in medium size or large towns (Piperno 1986), 82 % of interviewed declared that they had consulted a doctor (a specialist or a general practitioner) in the preceding year, with an average number of visits of 6.3: this figure corresponds to the results of the ISTAT survey, despite of the fact that the two studies concerned different sections of the populations and different periods of the year.

6. ACCOUNTING

The information needed to handle the administrative aspects of the doctor-patient-NHS relationship is collected by the USL. It is organized in regional or USL's computerized information systems (depending on the regional political attitude towards decentralization and on the computer architecture chosen). A minimum set of data concerning the doctor (identification, date of academic degree, number of practices and their addresses) and the patient (identification, date of birth, identification of the g.p. chosen, date of choice, date of eventual revoke) is required to calculate periodically the remuneration due to each doctor and to control that all inhabitants are correctly enrolled in the NHS.

However, in some regions the organization of such an information system was considered to be a too much complex and expensive undertaking, and (by an agreement with the g.p.s' representatives) a unique capitation fee has been fixed, depending on the age distribution of the whole population. In other cases, the information system finds it hard to become functioning, and the payment is still based on the doctor's declaration of the number of patients he has in his list (without any supporting documentation).

Therefore, the responsibility to authenticate the eligibility of patients and to collect the documentation needed for accounting is of the USL: the doctor can keep his list of patients if he wants (and all doctors do it, in fact), in order to control that payments have been made correctly; concerning his administrative relationship with the USL, he has only to prepare a list of all the 'extra' services that he has eventually provided to his patients, and the annual declaration of expenditures made which is mentioned in paragraph 4.

7. MEDICAL DOCUMENTATION

The NHS creation Act establishes that every USL should give to its inhabitants a Personal Health Booklet that the citizen is asked to hold; the USL should also care for the compilation and updating of this document. Following this Act, the Ministry of Health should have defined a unique model of Booklet, to be adopted by all the USLs. The last Contract of general practitioners mentions that the g.p.s should compile the booklets of their patients (on the USL's request) and should receive a remuneration for this function. The same Contract establishes that every doctor is charged to organize and to compile an individual Health Card for every patient, which is of his personal use.

However, the booklet's structure has never been defined by the Department of Health, because it was not clear whether the information collected could be actually handled for clinical and epidemiological purposes, with the reduced NHS's means, and because some risks of misuse have been foreseen (e.g. discrimination of a citizen with a history of ill health in the access to work).

Two years ago, the FIMG has proposed to his affiliates a model of Health Card. Besides the management of the clinical aspects concerning the individual patient, its objective was to collect morbidity data on specific problems to be defined each year: e.g. arterial hypertension, maternity and abortion, etc. This information could be made available to the central level of the NHS, for a computer processing of these data, aimed at giving a picture of problems of particular relevance to the planning and control activity.

This proposal has not been put into effect: but the need to define a common standard for the individual Health Card, following the principle of a 'Minimum Basic Data Set' to be collected with uniform criteria by all doctors (Lambert 1982), is recognized as being of great importance. Some USLs have adopted the model proposed by the FIMG; other Regions have designed their own models; others have limited their initiative to the definition of a ticket for the newborns, which contains only few data: identification of the citizen, its regional health code, g.p.'s regional code, blood group, ...).

The Department of Health has, among its projects, the objective to propose a modification of the article of the Law which mentions the booklet, to establish that every citizen should have:

(i) a Health Ticket with only few identification data, to be used for administrative purposes (including the choice of the doctor, the supply of drugs, the admission into the hospital, etc.);

(ii) a more detailed Health Card that the District should organize and handle for its inhabitants, primarily for epidemiological purposes.

In this project, the initiative concerning the doctor's record is left to the decision of the doctor himself and of his professional organizations.

8. ORGANIZATIONS AND PROFESSIONAL BODIES

Every graduate in medicine who wants to practice the medical profession has to enroll in the Medical Association (Ordine dei Medici). The Association is an 'auxiliary organization' of the State, as it is officially charged to represent the physicians in all peer committees which are involved in the application of the Contract. The Association is also charged to prepare, together with the Regional Consulting Committees, projects of professional training which have to be approved by the Region.

Various associations have been created to care for the professional interests of doctors: the Federation of General Practitioners (FIMG) with his 37 thousand associates, assists about 36 % of the g.p.s who have a contract with the NHS, and also many doctors who are not yet in the NHS's lists.

The Society of General Practitioners (SIMG) is a cultural association which corresponds to the Royal College of General Practitioners (Levitt 1979); it is a direct emanation of the FIMG and has been created to promote initiatives of permanent professional training. It publishes a revue which is sent to all g.p.s and organizes, in particular, a sector dedicated to informatics.

9. STATUS OF COMPUTER SUPPORT IN THE COUNTRY

The market of small computers is in a great rise in Italy: following the results of an inquiry by the Association of Industries of Informatics, about 600 thousand small computers had been sold, at the end of 84, for a value of 300 billions of lire (with an increase of 80 % from 83).

Many software products exist which are specially oriented to the general practitioner: they cover administrative aspects (accounting, booking of consultations, issuing of certificates and prescriptions) as well as clinical aspects (recording of history and therapy data, usually in predefined format).

However, these products are the result of craftsman-works frequently made by doctors who have a software agency: therefore, they do not respond to a serious analysis of requirements, and did not have much success among the g.p.s: the SIMG considers that not more than 200 doctors have a computer to assist them in their work.

An important thrust to this sector has been given by the Project of Informatics, which was promoted in 1981 by the National Research Council (CNR): this Project involved universities and other research institu tions, as well as private companies. In particular, a first project on the information system of the general practitioner was initiated, with the participation of the SIMG. The prototype that was produced on Olivetti M20 computers has not entered the market, but was a point of departure for other initiatives, oriented at producing commercial products.

Among them, it is noteworthy a project promoted by the SIMG to develop a modular system for personal computers with hard disk, which adopts a problem-oriented record, to integrate various functions of record keeping, production of certificates and prescriptions, statistics, lists of at-risk patients: the 'Classification of diseases, problems and procedures' of the Royal College of General Practitioners is used for coding diseases and problems. This product is going to be finished at the beginning of next year, and will be tested in various practices, before being made generally available. In particular, a research project in cooperation by the CNR and the Region of Liguria is aimed to test this prototype within a group of selected physicians, with special emphasis on the possibility of using clinical records for epidemiological purposes.

The main obstacle to the penetration of these systems into the market is that, notwithstanding what the Contract dictates, most doctors usually do not have a Health Card or a clinical record for their patients (50 and 60 % respectively, following the results of an inquiry on a sample of 300 physicians in the Region of Puglia: de Rosis 1985); therefore, they have to learn and to practice how to collect and to organize clinical information on their patients on paper records, first of all. But, besides this difficulty, there are also problems of financial nature: doctors should be incentivated, somehow, to devolve part of the allowance for practice expenses they receive from the NHS (in absence of any control and therefore as a fixed part of their remuneration) to the purchase of a computer and of the relative software. In a situation where they do not even keep a record for their patients, it is probable that no computer system will be sufficiently attractive to insure them a convenient cost/benefit ratio.

10. TRENDS AND FUTURE DEVELOPMENTS

The results of system analysis suggest some cues to the definition of programmes in this field:

(i) <u>which general practitioners</u> may have an interest in computerized information systems:

- those who are full-time g.p.s, and have a sufficient number of patients (at least 1000) and a sufficient remuneration, to require a rationalization of their work and information system, having at the same time the possibility to devolve part of their income to this objective. As in these cases the doctor has also a nurse who helps him in administrative and reception duties, he could entrust her with some input/output procedures. However, the initial organization of a file of 1000 - 1500 records implies a number of organizational and economical problems which probably need a greater professional advice and help than just selling an ad hoc software.

- those who have a second part-time work (as specialists or in a hospital) and therefore a reduced number of patients as g.p.s but, usually, a higher overall income; these doctors may have more experience in clinical record keeping, and therefore the organization of a computerized system could be easier to them. However, they need to organize files of different content and with different objectives for their diversified patients, and frequently cannot rely on a secretarial help.

- those young doctors who practice in groups, and who reach a reasonable income. In this case, a file for each doctor has to be organized, but everyone should also have the possibility to access the file of a colleague, and epidemiological analyses should be performed on the whole of files. This perspective is considered as one of the most promising for computerizing primary care practices: however, it is obviously conditioned to an extention of the present number of group practices, as a result of promotion initiatives from the NHS.

(ii) which are the priorities in the application fields:

- due to the system of remuneration and accounting adopted, clinical aspects are of higher interest than administrative ones. The possibility to obtain (as a byproduct of the record updating) prescriptions, certificates and notifications of infectious diseases on ad hoc forms is certainly needed, whereas the booking of consultations is a secondary objective: practices are generally open in fixed 'access hours', when the patients are allowed to enter and are visited with a criterium of 'first-in-first-out'. Due to the extremely brief duration of consultations in the ambulatory and due to the existance of domiciliary visits, any updating of computer files should probably be postponed after the daily closing of the practice: therefore, paper and magnetic records are going to coexist, at least until a reorganization of the practice work has been made, as an unavoidable byproduct of initiatives of computerization. A special solution has to be found for those doctors who have two practices (usually, in different USLs in the same city).

- the interest, for a g.p., to make epidemiological studies is, in the majority of cases, linked to being involved in initiatives of the USL, of the Region or of scientific institutions: only in exceptional cases, g.p.s who are not working in other facilities undertake a research work. However, the need to organize regularly initiatives of this kind is mentioned in the Contract and in the National Health Plan, and could contribute to break the isolation of g.p.s and to improve the present information on the population's health status and problems;

- the possibility to have a guide to the decision-making process is of undoubted importance, specially considering the limited age and experience of most of our g.p.s. However, one should consider that the large majority of problems that a doctor has to face in his activity are not serious,and that the serious problems he meets are extremely variable: therefore, the consultation system should not deal with rare and complex diseases, but should include protocols of action for common problems (see, e.g., the administration of drugs, which is a sector where the doctor receives presently no other information than the industrial advertizing).

As an example of the levels of priority that g.p.s assign to various possible functions of computerized information systems, see Table 6, which shows results of the inquiry already mentioned in paragraph 9 (de Rosis 1985).

Table 6. Levels of priorities in the possible functions of computerized medical records, as seen by doctors. Source: de Rosis 1985.

functions	levels of priority (in % of answers)		
	high	medium	low
rapid retrieval and updating of history and treatment	68	27	5
information on use, toxicity and effects of drugs	64	32	4
lists of at-risk patients	61	32	7
aid to diagnosis	57	29	14
therapeutic protocols	56	33	11
<u>printout of</u>:			
notifications of inf.diseases	44	44	12
request of specialist advice	38	49	13
prescription of drugs	35	50	15
certificates	34	50	16
subsections of the record	23	51	26
<u>statistical analysis</u> oriented to:			
evaluate efficacy of interventions	43	43	14
analyse the catchment area	38	40	22
measure the volumes of activity	39	38	23
<u>aid to administrative functions</u> like:			
booking of consultations	10	20	70
budgeting	8	40	52
control of payments by the USL	9	47	44

(iii) <u>which measures could favour the computerization</u> of g.p.s' practices:

- an interesting financial incentive could result from the FIMG's proposal for the new Contract, which demands to condition the maximum allowance for the expenses to the 'standard' of practices: this standard should be defined on the basis of the personnel and the instrumentations being in the practice itself, the presence of a computer being a parameter that should contribute to increase the standard at its maximum.

- a real encouragement for group practices should be given by the NHS, particularly for those young doctors who have a professional interest to this kind of work: the incentives required concern the possibility to use an ambulatory in common with public primary care services, and to have a nursing and a secretarial help partially paid by the NHS.

REFERENCES

Berlinguer G, de Rosis F (1983) Balance sheet of health organization reform in Italy. Effective Health Care 1:143-152
de Rosis F, Ricci FL, Rossi Mori A (1984) Prescrizioni di farmaci: un sistema informativo mirato ad obiettivi di intervento. Prospettive Sociali e Sanitarie 7:9-12
de Rosis F, D'Ercole M (1985) Indagine sul sistema informativo dei medici di base in Puglia. Internal Report ISI
Greco M, Boni M (1982) La disciplina dei rapporti con i medici di medicina generale convenzionati con le USL. Ragno, Roma 178
ISTAT (1984) Indagine statistica sulle condizioni di salute della popolazione e sul ricorso ai servizi sanitari. Notiziario ISTAT 4
Lambert PM, Roger FH (1982) Hospital Statistics in Europe. North Holland Amsterdam p 200
Levitt R (1979) The reorganized National Health Service. Redwood Burn Ltd, London p 254
Ministero della Sanità (1984) Relazione sullo stato sanitario del Paese 1980. Istituto Poligrafico dello Stato, Roma, p 365
Ministero della Sanità, Servizio Centrale della Programmazione Sanitaria (1985). Flussi informativi delle USL. Internal Report.
Panti A (1985) Inchiesta: quello che pensa il medico di famiglia. Il medico d'Italia, 3:35
Piperno A, Renieri A (1981) Il comportamento del medico generico in Italia. Prospettive Sociali e Sanitarie 9: 23-35
Piperno A (1986) La politica sanitaria in Italia. F Angeli, Milano,p 375
Splendori F, Vanini G (1985) Censimento dei medici italiani al 30.6.1984. Supp. to La Rivista Medica Italiana, p 452

ACKNOWLEDGEMENTS

Most of data and information used in this analysis results from informal discussions with experts in this sector and unpublished documentation. The author is specially obliged to the Servizio Centrale della Programmazione Sanitaria, Department of Health, and to the Secretary General of the FIMG, for their kind help.

ONE OR TWENTY-SIX HEALTH CARE SYSTEMS IN SWITZERLAND?

Dr. A. Assimacopoulos

Division d'Informatique, Hôpital Cantonal Universitaire,
CH-1211 Genève 4/Switzerland

INTRODUCTION

Switzerland is a federation of 26 states and semi-states having their own autonomy. A few major questions such as defense, foreign affairs, custom, money, transportation and telecommunication have been delegated by the cantons to the federal state. But many other questions are remaining at the level of the cantons (our states) with very little influence of the federal level on these questions. Among these questions there is police, laws, education and health care.

The time of the year at which the school year begins is a good example of the autonomy of the cantons. In Bern or Zurich, two of the largest states, the school year starts at Easter, whereas in many other cantons such as Geneva or Basel the school year starts in August or mid-September.

This federalism, namely a different solution for each state, is also well present in the field of health care or public health. Two federal laws are drawing the general frame work of the Swiss health care system. The first law deals with health care insurances for diseases and for the protection of motherhood. The second law prescribes mandatory health care insurances for injuries due to accidents in employed persons.

This differentiation between diseases and injuries is of importance since different regulations are in effect for these two types of medical situations. Any medical event has to be classified by the physician. According to the judgement: accident or disease, a different third party will be selected: It will be either one of the numerous health care mutual insurances in case of disease, or one of the also numerous insurance companies for injuries.

1. STRUCTURE OF PRIMARY CARE

1.1. Who delivers primary care?

Due to the weak impact of federal regulations on local laws nearly all imaginable types of medical organisation can be find in Switzerland. Nevertheless, a clear-cut distinction has to be made between privately offered and state offered health care. In-patient health care is traditionally delivered by public or state operated hospitals; ambulatory care (on the opposite) is offered mainly by private practitioners or institutions.

In spite of a few exceptions, private practices or health centers have no links with hospitals. The structure of a building housing doctor's offices on one side of a street with a large hospital on the other is unfrequent.

The density of private practitioners is high in our country. There was one practitioner for 816 inhabitants in 1980 with a clear trend towards augmentation. But this density is definitively not homogeneous, in rural countries such as the canton of Uri there is one physician for 1470 inhabitants, whereas the proportion is one for 500 in the city of Basel.

The private practices are generally opened at office hours. Some physicians open their offices early in the morning or late in the afternoon. Round-the-clock services can be obtained either through a few private or public group practices or through the local medical association. Indeed their members frequently participate by rotation in an on-call service.

Home visits are exceptional in urban areas, but seem to remain frequent in rural areas or in mountains. In these areas, physicians can spent 3 to 5 hours a day visiting their patients at home.

The number of specialists is high, two specialists for each generalist (general practitioner). But this figure has to be commented. Many specialists for internal medicine are in fact general practitioners. This situation has been created on purpose by an important difference in the prices specialists are allowed to charge. These high revenues keep physicians back from opening their private practice the day following their graduation from medical school and encourage them towards post-graduate training. Little more than a decade ago the Swiss Medical Association (Federatio Medicorum Helveticorum - FMH) created a title of specialist in general practice with a proper curriculum. Aside from young doctors completing their post-graduate training in hospitals the number of full-time hospital physicians is extremely low. Two elements can explain this situation:

- Two third of the medical staff in large hospitals are physicians completing their curriculum of specialists during 5, 8 or 10 years, and then shall open their own private practice.

- The remaining third is the permanent hospital medical staff. Most of these physicians have a part-time (half a day to one full day weekly) private ambulatory practice.

For example, in Geneva, among 850 fully trained physicians around 50 are full-time hospital staff members.

1.2. Personnel

In 1980, about 150.000 persons were employed in the field of health care. This mean 5.2 percent of the active population. Most of them were hospital employees (4 percent of the active population). A typical ambulatory practice is made of one physician and a (full-time or part-time) receptionist. This person (usually a female) is either a clerk or a former nurse or someone with a specific training for the profession. She is in charge of most of the clerical tasks and has some technical skill such as laboratory or radiology. Specialists employ more technical personnel. In Geneva for example 440 practitioners employ 1319 persons (physician and part-time employee included) (Cresson-Steinauer, 1985). The wife of the physician is frequently a part-time employee of the practice.

Biology laboratories, pharmacists, physical therapists, opticians, psychologists and other paramedical professionals are generally available through private practice. It can be noted that in a few cantons physicians are also allowed to sell drugs due to the low density of population in their area.

The field of home care nursing is under expansion. These services are generally provided by private or public foundations trying to provide social services for people in need. The availability of such services in the different parts of Switzerland is uneven.

1.3. Expenditures

The Swiss population (6.3 millions) spends 14.500 millions of Swiss Francs yearly for their health. 46 percent of this money goes for the hospitals, 19.5 percent goes for private physicians, 8.7 percent for drugs, and 9.7 percent for dental care.

The yearly gross income of a physician is 370.000 SFr. Running costs are generally estimated as 50 to 65 percent of this income (state taxes excluded). The taxes rate for this income is about 30 percent.

Each family spends 6 to 7 percent of their income for medical and health care.

These figures will vary between cantons.

2. CATCHMENT AREAS, MOBILITY OF CHOICE

The liberty of choosing a physician is one important element in the Swiss health care system. Everybody is allowed to choose any physician practicing in his area. Two elements are somewhat moderating this statement:

- Practicing medicine in one of the cantons requires a federal diploma of physician and an authorisation from the local Ministry of Health. This authorisation is valid only within the canton where it has been delivered. Therefore, if a patient from one canton is visiting a physician from an other canton, the rate of remuneration for the medical acts will be that of the canton where the patient is living.

- For chronically ill patients or invalids insured by the federal insurance for invalidity moving from one physician to another one must be authorised by the insurance, in order to have the costs of treatment covered by the insurance.

Practically, the patients are selecting physicians either in the village or neighborhood where they are living, and sometimes where they are working.

Young adults have a tendency to visit health centers offering permanent services and a rotation of physicians. But when they are becoming around 45 or 50 years old they start to have a stable general practitioner.

Any patient can make an appointment with any specialist such as dermatologist, surgeon, cardiologist at any time. A preliminary visit with a generalist is neither compulsory nor required by the health insurances. But some specialists ask their patients to be first visited by a generalist.

The number of old persons is increasing regularly each year. People over 65 represent around 14 percent of the total population.

According to the health insurance organisations, treatments take place within periodes of three months or any multiple of three.

Any disease exceeding 720 days of consecutive illness is considered as a chronic disease. It implies a modification in the coverage status by the insurance.

3. STRUCTURE OF PRACTICES AND USAGES

The largest majority of physicians is practicing their art in single practice. But studies on group-practice indicated a tendency towards an increase of group-practice. The mean age of the physicians involved in group-practice is below the average of the medical population(Cresson-Steinhauer, 1985).

In Geneva, among 640 practitioners in 1980, 47 were practicing in 12 groups. In the German speaking part of our country 203 groups were recorded, 72 percent of them were associations of two physicians, 18 percent of three physicians. In addition to the growing number of this type of practice, group-practice per se is a potential market for computer applications.

The associations can be divided in three classes:

- Equipment sharing: the personnel is hired by each physician separately, accounting is separate, only some equipments and rooms are shared.
- Practice groups: the equipments, the rooms and the personnel are shared between the physicians. Accounting is separate, only the collective expenses are divided among the participating physicians either on a fixed rate or on a rate adjusted to the use of a particular facility by each physician.
- Grouped practice: all equipment, personnel income and expenses are shared.

The first two types are the most frequent ones (37 and 40 percent respectively of all group-practices). The generalists and internists are present in this type of association at a high frequency when compared with the overall medical population. Surgeons and orthopedists are also rather frequent.

4. REMUNERATION

The major distinction made in the introduction of this paper between insurances for diseases and for accidents has a large impact on all the financial questions. The remuneration for services in ambulatory practice is always made according to the quantity and the nature of services. But the list of services and their prices vary from one canton to another and may also vary according to the type of insurance covering the patient.

The major classes of insurances are:

- mutual insurances for diseases,
- federal insurances,
- private insurances for accidents or supplement coverage in case of disease.

4.1. Principles of remuneration

The principles of remuneration are different for each type of insurance.

4.1.1. Mutual insurances for diseases

These insurances are extremely numerous in Switzerland (more than 500). They are operating under a federal law giving the general rules for this type of insurance. According to the regulations in the various cantons, insurances either are reimbursing the bill to the patient or are paying the bill directly to the physicians (third party payer).

In each canton an agreement is made periodically between the local federation of mutual insurances, the local medical association and the local Ministry of Health in order to determine the list of acts that are covered by the insurance and mainly their prices.

The physicians agree to write their bills according to this list, and the insurances to pay the bills up to 90 percent of the total. The difference (10 percent) is paid by the patient himself.

This system means that not only the price of each act may change any time, but also that the list of acts and its classification is subject to modifications. These modifications will be more than just cosmetic. In spite of the fact that this insurance is not mandatory, 97 percent of the population are covered by this type of mutual insurances.

4.1.2. Federal insurances

There are only three federal insurances, the national insurance against accidents (CNA-SUVA), the federal military insurance (AMF), and the insurance for invalids (AI-IV). These insurances, covering a minority of cases, are always paying the bills directly to the physicians. The list of medical acts, their classification and prices are rather homogeneous among these three insurances.

The lists of acts accepted for billing and their prices are generally determined by the federal office for social insurances (OFAS). This list of acts could be the origin of a national standard, but it is presently limited to injuries. No standard exists for disease insurances. The first insurance of this section (CNA) is compulsory for certain categories of employees (construction and factories' workers). The coverage includes any kind of accidents and the professional diseases.

4.1.3. Private insurances

The private insurances are either covering the costs due to accidents or are offering extra coverage to some services that are not covered by the mutual insurances (i.e. hospitalisation in private hospital instead of a public one, etc.)

The list of procedures and prices is generally that of the federal office for social insurances, but this is only true for situations covered by the federal law for accident insurances. The bill is generally addressed to the patient as for mutual insurances for disease.

Since January 1985 the basic insurance for accidents became compulsory for every employee.

4.2. Surveillance

No detailed rules for surveillance are in effect. The insurances appoint physicians to review cases for unusual situations or abuses. In a few cantons the local federation of mutual insurances are pooling their expenses for each of the private practitioners. The physicians generating greater cost per case than average are put under pressure by the insurances to reduce their costs. This raises a question: should this be done by the insurances or by a peer review group?

The physicians appointed by the insurances are generally private practitioners, except for federal insurances where few physicians are employed.

5. STRUCTURE OF PATIENTS

The mutual insurances are covering 66 percent of the total expenses in ambulatory care. The part paid by the federal insurances is estimated to be around 3 percent of these expenses. The private insurances of the patients themselves are paying the remaining part.

In primary care, aside of university medical centers and hospitals, there are no proper ambulatory centers for special type of patients. The only specialisation observed is due to the medical specialities.

A tendency can nevertheless be observed towards a better handling of elderly persons. Will this lead to the creation of specialised ambulatory centers for this type of patients? The question remains open.

6. ACCOUNTING

No diagnosis is required for accounting. The only justification is the description of the accident in case of services to be paid by an insurance of this type. The bills sent by the physician to the patient indicate always the grand total and a list of codes relating to the various visits, procedures or treatments. The code book is different from one type of insurance to the other and differs also among cantons for the branch of mutual insurances. For example, the white blood cells counts might include the differential count in one list of codes, but may not include it in the other. Moreover, its relative price may change from one year to the other. Every diagnostic or therapeutic procedure performed by a non-physician has to be ordered by a physician in order to be covered by the insurance.

6.1. Time and structure of accounting

The duration of treatment is defined by the structure of the federal law governing mutual insurances. The periodicity of billing is of three months. The habit has therefore been taken that the bill will be sent three months after the first visit, but this is only a habit, and not a rule. This period of three months is the validity duration of a so-called "disease sheet" issued by the insurance on the request of a patient.

Any treatment lasting longer than 720 days exceeds the limits of coverage for mutual insurance. The patient is supposed to be an invalid and is possibly entitled to receive coverage by the federal insurance for invalids.

A certificate of insurance is distributed to patients by the insurances. But in ambulatory practice neither this certificate nor the so-called "disease sheet" issued by the insurance is of any use since the bill is generally addressed to the patient.

6.2. Processing of claims

The pharmacist is generally sending his bills directly to the mutual insurances. He is using a copy of the "disease sheet" to determine the end of the three months period. Physicians working under the system of the third party payer use a similar mechanism.

The claims are processed by the insurances and the payments will be made either to the patient, the doctor or the pharmacist. The 10 percent of the bill corresponding to the contribution of the patient to the cost of his disease will be requested from the patient by the insurance for all the bills paid directly by the insurance to the provider of services.

7. MEDICAL DOCUMENTATION

As far as private practice is concerned no legal rules are existing for medical documentation. Some constraints are induced by legal requirements for accounting, reporting of some infectious diseases and tumors. It is suggested that physicians are maintaining patient files where they record important information on the patient. No description of these files is included in the law. It is not clear presently whether these files belong, at least in some way, to the patient or whether they are to be considered as a private note booklet belonging to the physician.

The legal requirements are dealing as already mentioned with accounting and with drug prescriptions. In order to be reimbursed by the insurance, any drug given to a patient has to be ordered on a document signed by a physician authorise to practise in the canton. Moreover some drugs can be obtained only upon presentation of a drug prescription.

These elements are extremely positive for the development of computerised systems for the ambulatory practice.

8. GOVERNMENTAL AND NON-GOVERNMENTAL ORGANISATIONS

In addition to the departments of public health and medical associations of each of the 26 cantons and semi-cantons, it is important to quote some federal offices: such as the federal office for social insurances, the Swiss national insurance for accidents, and the Swiss Association for Hospitals (VESKA) because of their influence on the definition of procedures and their classification.

A comprehensive list of all these associations, offices and organisations, and of all the physicians, dentists and pharmacists is published yearly. It is a key to every component of the Swiss health system (quoted under references).

The Swiss Medical Informatics Society (SSIM) has been created this spring. It has not yet been active in the field of ambulatory care. But the growing number of physicians considering the acquisition of computer services for their own practice will create pretty soon a need for a survey of this market, pooling good and bad experiences and promoting some standards in the field of type of services, quality, performance and prices.

9. STATUS OF COMPUTER SUPPORT IN SWITZERLAND

9.1. Penetration

The Swiss market is extremely open to computers of any size: giant ones, large ones and PCs. Probably each manufacturer is present in this market. Many software or tailor-made products are available, but the average survival time of the houses supporting them is questionable.

In spite of a good penetration of the market in general, the medical field has been very reluctant and probably still is rather reluctant towards computers. The fact that Switzerland is the second last European country to have created a national society for medical informatics is probably the indication of a circumspect approach towards medical informatics. No census is available of the number of computers installed in the field of ambulatory care.

In Geneva, around 5 percent of the private practitioners have a computer or are using the services of a computer for the accounting. For example, a physician, considering the use of a private computer for his practice, received 7 proposals for a system. The proposals came from independent vendors, five of them were interested in the development of a system. One had recently installed a tailor-made system for a few physicians in another canton and proposed some alterations for the local needs. One of the vendors was in negotiation with a constructor in order to have his software taken over by the company. None of the bids came from large companies.

9.2. Type of systems

The majority of systems available for private practices are purely dedicated to accounting.

At first, off-line systems have been offered as pooled services for accounting and billing. The introduction of PCs opens the market for on-line multipurpose systems. The main benefit of computers remains accounting, but modules are proposed for drug prescription, medical certificates, incorporated word processors, medical statistics and also medical records. The availability of such systems is too recent (one or two years) to assess the rate of usage of the various modules. But a fully automated system for the ambulatory practice is said to be commercially available in the main areas of our country.

9.3. Problems

In addition to the problems attached to the computer technology itself, such as:

- rapid turnover of hardware and software,
- lack of stability of vendors in the field of dedicated applications,
- lack of experience of conversion from one system to another,
- etc.,

two particular problems are existing for Switzerland. The first is the variety of rules existing between the cantons and between the types of insurances. This diversity of rules induces rather complex solutions even within one canton in order to allow the physician to evolve with his system from one set of rules to another one the next year.

The second major problem might come from the data security laws presently under preparation in our country. Some cantons have already data security laws governing the relation of the individual with his local state. But the relation between individuals is a matter that has to be addressed by the federal laws. The federal law for data security will probably state that a person should be given access to his record. Depending on the way the medical record is considered, i.e. as a patient belonging or as a physician's private belonging, the use of computers in private ambulatory care might remain limited to accounting or evolve to total medical records.

10. CONCLUSION AND FUTURE TRENDS

Up to now, a lot of attention has been paid to medical care as delivered by hospitals. This is adequate since costs of hospitals are the largest part of the total expences for public health (46 percent in our country). But ambulatory care represents another large part of these expenses: i.e. 41 percent in our country, including medical (19,5 percent) and dental (9,7 percent) care as well as drugs.

The introduction of computers in the field of ambulatory care should promote a better monitoring of the activity in this field. The evaluation should not only include financial questions, but also medical issues: Who are the patients visiting our ambulatory facilities? For what kind of complaints are they coming? Is the offered response adequate? Are we doing better with new treatments? etc.

Medical research in the primary care is underdeveloped when compared with the hospital based clinical research. Private practitioners should be appealed towards research programs in ambulatory care since in our country an important part of the patients are visiting exclusively privately operated primary care facilities. Computer applications could be used as a clinical data acquisition tool plugged into the day to day reality. But what type of information should be captured?; diagnosis, psychological complaints, acuteness and severity of complaints, risks, etc? A new metric needs probably to be invented for the monitoring of primary care.

REFERENCES

Cresson-Steinhauer, G. (1985): Cabinets médicaux de groupe à Genève, Ed.: Réalités sociales, Case postale 797, CH-1201 Lausanne.

Gygi, P., Frei, A. (1984): Das schweizerische Gesundheitswesen, G. Krebs AG, Basel.

Annuaire statistique 1984, Ed.: Service cantonal de la statistique, Département de l'économique publique, Genève.

Annuaire médical suisse, 1984, Ed.: Schwabe et Cie S.A., Basel.

STRUCTURE OF THE HEALTH SYSTEM AND PRACTICAL ASPECTS OF COMPUTER USE IN PRIMARY CARE

J. Zvárová, C. Dostal [+], V. Zámková

Department of Social Medicine, Medical Faculty, Charles University Prague, Czechoslovakia

+ Research Institute of Rheumatology, Prague

Introduction

In the Czechoslovak Socialist Republic human health is the cornerstone of the well-being and all-round development of every individual, but also a significant factor of economic and social progress. The inalienable right of every individual to health is not only proclaimed but translated into practice. Already the Constitution of 9th May 1948 guaranteed to all citizens the right of health protection, medical treatment and social security in old age or in a case of incapacity for work, to women the right of a special care in pregnancy and maternity, to children and young adolescent people the right of the insurance of a full physical and mental development (Hořejší, 1982). The unification of the whole health service came about in 1952, when the Act of the unified preventive and medical care came into force and the bill on hygienic and epidemiologic services was passed. Thanks to these historic acts new organizations entered our health services such as the district system, health centers for out-patients related to hospital care, regional arrangements of medical institutions, the creation of organizational complexes of national health institute and of organs of hygienic and epidemiologic services.

By the historic act "On the People's Health Care", which was adopted in 1966 and is still valid, Czechoslovakia became the first country in the world to pay all its citizens from their birth to death all costs of health care, including medicaments and even the most expensive curative procedures. We read in its preamble: "Health is one of the basic preconditions of a happy and creative life of an individual as well as of the whole society; it is also a significant agent in the development of productive forces. The efforts to attain the best possible health are therefore one of the main tasks of a socialist society."

Schools and postgraduate institutes are by far not the only ones which help doctors and other workers in health service to broaden their knowledge and keep abreast of the dynamic progress of medicine. We want to mention also the Czechoslovak Medical Society J.E. Purkyně.

The Czechoslovak Medical Society J.E. Purkyně is composed of 54 specialized societies and of the Physicians Associations in 42 Czech and 37 Slovak towns; today the basis of the Czechoslovak Medical Society is formed by more than 29.000 physicians, by over 3.000 pharmacists and by nearly 16.000 paramedical workers and nurses.

Nowadays, from many aspects the modern socialist health service is a quite new quality with which we can only with much difficulty compare not only our past, but also the present reality in a number of other countries.

Structure of primary health care

The basis of specialized medical care provided by a system of health establishments in Czechoslovakia are the community primary medical services. These are available in territorial or enterprise-based (works) health care communities, which represent an integrated part of the whole area under the respective hospital with a policlinic or a policlinic outside the hospital (Graph 1).

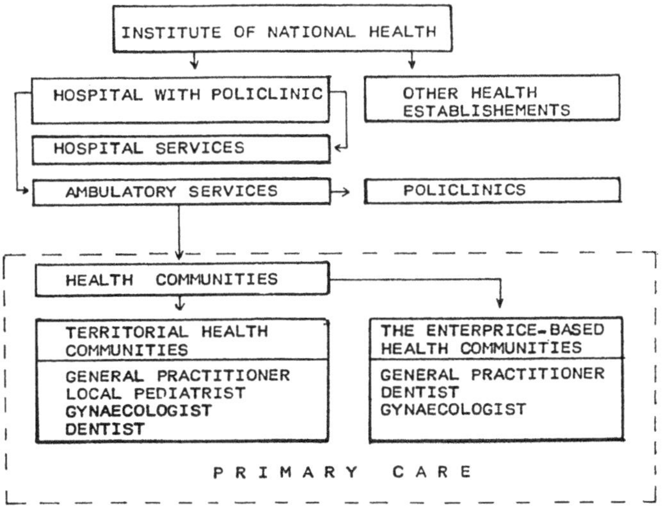

Similarly to the whole system of health care services, these communal services have a regional structure. The health care community is a precisely defined territorial region (or an enterprise) where the population living or working in a given area enjoys health care services provided by a group of (para-)medical staff under the supervision and leadership of the local general practitioner. The territory belonging to this health care community is an integral part of the area under the authority of a hospital with a policlinic, or a policlinic outside the premises of the hospital. In this way the organizational relation between the communal system and the system of hospitals and policlinics is secured.

The essential purpose of communal health services is to provide basic out-patient health care to the population, and apart from tasks in the process health education, hygiene and the struggle against contagious diseases, it should also mediate further specialized health care. They should be in charge of active preventive health check-ups, providing in cooperation with the specialized policlinic and hospital departments continuous dispensary care to the selected groups of the population. These services are to be made available either directly in the patient's home, or wherever else it may be necessary.

Territorial health communities include the general practitioner, the local pediatrist, gynaecologist and dentist. The medical nurse, gynaecologist's nurse, a nurse in charge of elderly and chronically ill patients, instrument nurse or the dentist's laboratory assistant and the ambulance driver if in exceptional cases the car is under the authority of the local health community, they all provide the necessary health services. These services are available for population living in a given region, or working in selected small enterprises. Furthermore, these services are available for people regularly commuting to work, school or people who for any other similar reason, due to excessive loss of time cannot use the local facilities where they live. However, permanent health care can be provided for these people only in special cases and with the approval of the general practitioner territorially assigned to the patient. Finally the territorial communal health care services are also available for those citizens who live in another territory and yet have chosen this particular practitioner and obtained his approval.

In an enterprise-based health care community, the services include the general practitioner, the dentist or a gynaecologist. Members of the medical staff further include: the medical nurse, gynaecologist's nurse, dentist's instrument nurse or a medical nurse to the local dentist and the dentist's laboratory assistant. The staff of the enterprise health community centre provides its services for the employees of the enterprise (or its particular part or several enterprises together). If it is an open enterprise-based health centre, it may also provide health care services for selected groups of people (e.g. family members, former employees, inhabitants of housing estate nearby, etc.). These services may also include the visiting medical practitioner.

The territorial health community is located either in the local health centre (covering one or several communities) or the local policlinic.
The enterprise-based health community is located either in the enterprise health centre (with one or several communities) or the enterprise health station or as enterprise policlinic. In exceptional cases the enterprise health community may be located in the territorial health establishment.

There is a long-term trend towards the concentration of city health communities into policlinics and in rural areas into communal health care centers covering two or more communities and such establishments are now being built in larger villages. In spite of this trend, in order to make health care available to the population living in remote parts of the country, sometimes with difficult access, the establishing of health care stations, pediatric and gynaecological consulting bureaus is possible, functioning as advanced facilities of the communal health centres. In exceptional cases health care may be provided in these localities by means of mobile facilities. The territories and locations of health care communities are defined by the District National Committee on the basis of a proposal of the district Institute of National Health and in cooperation with local National Committee (for territorial communities) or trade unions (for enterprise-based communities) in accordance with principles formulated by the Ministry of Health.

The numbers of establishments of out-patient curative and preventive care and several indicators of our health care system are given in Table 1. /Historical statistical year-book 1985/.

Table 1 : ESTABLISHMENTS OF OUT-PATIENT CURATIVE AND PREVENTIVE CARE IN CZECHOSLOVAKIA TO 31. 12. 1983

Type	Poli-clinics	Community health centres	Medical stations	Consultation rooms for women	children	Total	Doctors absol.	posts No. per one policlinic
TERRITORIAL	380	1842	778	66	2 287	5 353	22584.9	59.43
IN WORKS +	54	1118	1580	-	-	2 753	5505.84	101.96

(+ including Czechoslovak State Railways)

The employees of the Czechoslovak health care institutions are divided into groups of specialized medical staff and non-medical professions, and further into various categories and specializations (Table 2).

Table 2 : DOCTOR'S POSTS IN HEALTH CARE ESTABLISHEMENTS IN CZECHOSLOVAKIA TO DECEMBER 31st 1983

TYPE OF ESTABLISHMENT	DOCTOR´S POSTS NUMBER	%	FOR 10 000 INHABITANTS
GENERAL HOSPITALS AND MATERNITY HOMES +	10 904	24.3	7.06
ESTABLISHMENTS OF OUT-PATIENT CURATIVE AND PREVENTIVE CARE	28 090	62.6	18.31
ESTABLISHMENTS OF HEALTH SERVICES IN TOTAL	44 880	100.0	29.11

+ including Czechoslovak State Railways

Table 3 shows the proportions of individual groups and categories in selected types of health care establishments.

Table 4 shows the volume of activity in these territorial and enterprise-based health care communities, in proportion to the total activity of the whole out-patient curative and preventive care network.

Table 3: WORKERS IN SELECTED HEALTH CARE ESTABLISHMENTS BY CATEGORIES AND SELECTED ESTABLISHMENTS AND IN TOTAL (TO 31.12.1983)

Health establishment	Doctors	Pharmacists	Other workers +	Dentists ++	Paramed. personnel	Lower health pers.	Auxil. health pers.	Total +++	Others	Total
General and maternity hospitals	11.462 26.1%	9 0.2%	3 38.0%	399 9.7%	42.761 33.1%	1.576 17.7%	4.660 39.6%	60.870 30.0%	29.717 32.9%	90.587 30.9%
Establishm. of out-pat. curat. and prevent. care	26.490 60.2%	6 0.1%	1 13%	854	41.683 32.2%	2.989 33.5%	956 8.1%	72.929 35.9%	11.877 13.1%	84.806 28.9%
Total health establishm.	43.991 100%	5.235 100%	8 100%	4.101 100%	129.115 100%	8.926 100%	11.783 100%	203.159 100%	90.415 100%	293.574 100%

\+ other workers with university education in health care
++ other workers with professional school education in health care and dentists
+++ workers in health care total

Table 4 : NUMBER OF CONSULTATIONS (EXAMINATIONS) PERFORMED AND HOURS WORKED IN ESTABLISHMENTS OF OUT-PATIENT CURATIVE AND PREVENTIVE CARE

	NUMBER OF HOURS WORKED		NUMBER OF CONSULTATIONS AND EXAMINATIONS PERFORMED	
	Total	in %	Total	in %
TERRITORIAL AND WORKS FACILITIES -TOTAL	53 686 104	100.0	225 842 176	100.0
TERRITORIAL AND WORKS COMMUNITIES -DOCTORS	13 945 596	26.0	80 707 455	35.7

Health insurance

Health insurance of workers in Czechoslovakia is understood as an integral part of health care for the population.

Health insurance provides material security to workers temporarily out of work due to sickness, injury, quarantine, sickness in the family or pregnancy of working women. It also contributes by partially covering the cost connected with the birth of a child, education and nutrition of children not provided for otherwise as well as funeral in the family.

Basically, all citizens of Czechoslovakia are covered by the health insurance scheme. The insurance policy begins on the first day of employment and expires after the termination of the job. However, the worker is entitled to his insurance benefits also for a given time after that within the so-called "period of protection".

Health insurance is under the authority of the Revolutionary Trade Union Movement. This means that the trade unions not only decide about insurance benefits and supervise all financial transactions, but they also make sure (within preventive medical care) that conditions are created to decrease the sickness and mortality rate.

Insurance policy holders, including family members are entitled to insurance benefits.

A Czechoslovak citizens has a legal right of most of the insurance benefits. Some benefits are optional and the decision falls within the competence of the trade unions.

Insurance benefits are divided into financial and material:

1. Financial benefits
   - sickness allowance
   - contribution during the time of nursing of a sick family member
   - balance contribution in pregnancy and motherhood (when a women has to aspect a less paid job)
   - financial assistance in maternity
   - childbirth bonus

Health insurance also includes certain benefits for mother and child, in particular the maternity allowance incorporated in the legal system.

2. Material benefits
   - Spa treatment
   - Spa treatment in an optional benefit.

   Decisions of trade unions in this respect are guided by the medical urgency of the application and by the worker's professional merit.

Health insurance benefits in 1983 amounted to 28.799,0 million Czechoslovak crowns, i.e. 7 % of the national income.

References

Hořejší J. (1982) Zdraví pro 15 milionů, Avicenum, Praha

Historická statistická ročenka (1985) SNTL/ALFA, Praha

Primary health care system in Poland

J. Janecki

Doc. Dr. med. Jerzy Janecki, Samodzielna Pracownia Informatyki Kliniczney IBIB PAN, ul. Rutkowskiego 12, 00-020 Warszawa, PL

0. INTRODUCTION

The structure of health care in Poland differs considerably from such systems in many other European countries. In its majority it is based on National Health Care System of general access, but there are also private and cooperative ambulatories. Principally health care is of general access, but some governmental departments, i.e. the Department of National Defence, the Department of Justice, Home Office and the Department of Transport have their own health care systems.

The system of medical care of general access, for adults, controlled by the Minister of Health will be presented here. However, information concerning more general problems will be added whenever possible.

1. STRUCTURE OF PRIMARY CARE

1.1 General health care system consists of basic level, provincial level, hospitals of Medical Schools and Research Institutes, sanatoria, social care centers and pharmacies. Primary care is delivered by basic and partially by provincial level units.

The organizational units within the basic level are Integrated Health Care Centers (IHCC): ones of general access, occupational and for the highschools. Primary care is delivered mostly by district ambulatories, ambulatories within enterprises and universities (in urban areas) and by county, rural and enterprise based Health Centers (outside urban areas). On the provincial level the primary care is also delivered by ambulatories in some hospitals and by centers of Emergency Care.

1.2 In 376 Integrated Health Care Centers of general access, 40 Occupational and 8 Universitary Centers the primary care is delivered in outpatient clinics of general practice, pediatry and gynaecology. Among 69,231 Polish physicians 13,061 (18.9 %) are employed in primary care, which means 1 physician employed per 2,810 persons. In urban areas 9,303 physicians are employed in primary care (1 per 2,190 persons), in rural areas - only 3,758 physicians, hence 1 per 3,940 persons. The difference is due to greater number of pediatricians and gynaecologists in urban areas: 4,605 general practitioners are employed in urban areas, i.e. 1 per 4,750 persons and 3,094 in rural areas, i.e. 1 per 4,790. It has to be added that in 2,289 ambulatories within big industrial enterprises, almost exclusively urban, additional 3,932 general practitioners are employed. As in 344 industrial outpatient clinics for women there are also 742 physicians employed, it is obvious that the best primary care is delivered to women employed in industry and living in urban areas.

The numbers concerning physicians employed in primary care can be compared with 17,904 physicians employed in hospitals.

Among 186,944 nurses and midwives in Poland 27,262 (14.6 %) are employed in primary care; 17,877 in urban and 9,385 in rural areas. Especially many nurses are employed in pediatric and gynaecologic outpatient clinics in urban areas: while in general outpatient clinics the ratio of physicians to nurses is 1 : 1.56, in pediatrics it is 1 : 2.29 and in gynaecology 1 : 2.22. Nurses in primary care are supported by 21,869 Polish Red Cross sisters and 8,221 social care workers.

The quantitative relation between primary and specialistic care can be expressed by number of consultations per year: 79,625,575 in primary care clinics and 52,954,916 in specialistic ones. Pediatric care is the most intensive one: 40.5 % of all consultations in primary care were delivered to children.

In 1,494 district ambulatories 39 millions of consultations were delivered, including 5.4 millions (13.7 %) in outpatient clinics of 210 hospitals.

In primary care there are employed mainly general practitioners and internists (7,699), pediatricians (4,303) and gynaecologists (1,059). Generally, they are experienced physicians, middle aged, in 60 % specialists qualified in their respective fields.

1.3 Health care expenditures in 1983 amounted to 331,000 million zlotys, which corresponds to 5,3 % of National Revenue. Average monthly salary of a physician amounted that year to 16,226 zlotys, whereas the national average was 14,475 zlotys.

2. STRUCTURE OF POPULATION AND CATCHMENT AREAS

In 1983 Poland was inhabited by 36.7 million people: 18.8 million women (51.4 %) and 17.9 million men. Urban population amounted to 21.9 million (59.6 %), rural - 14.8 million.

21.66 million persons belonged to professionally active age groups (18-64 years for men and 18-59 years for women). Among them 11.1 million were men, 10.56 million were women.

There are no statistical data concerning disease incidence. Some insight into morbidity may be given by data concerning absence in work (in days) due to some frequent diseases:

Type of disease	days of absence (in millions)
total	181.1
acute pulmonary diseases	26.3
neural diseases	15.3
osseal-muscular diseases	13.1
pregnancy complications	10.9
cardio-vascular diseases	10.7
morbus ulcerosus	7.6
rheumatic arthritis	7.2
hypertension	6.8
neuroses	6.6
bronchitis and asthma	6.2

Each person has access to primary care in his district. Urban ambulatories are open for 9-12 hours daily. 24 hours' duties are performed by Emergency Care Units and in some large urban areas there are also systems of Night Medical Care, manned by primary care employees. Rural Health Centers are open accordingly to the working hours of medical staff employed.

The working hours of a physician employed in primary care are divided between consulting-hours and visits made at home (usually 4 and 3 hours respectively). A patient can fix an appointment at the registration desk of an ambulatory, his medical documentation is then transferred to his district physician. In cases of severe sickness, a patient can ask for a visit by telephone or through a third party. The visit will take place the same day and will be made by the district physician or his colleague from the same ambulatory or by a physician from Medical Night Care or, in urgent cases, by an Emergency Care physician.

Generally, the patient is directed to a physician caring for the patient's district. For the last two years a mobility of choice has been introduced, however, the change is slow and it is possible only where there are more general practitioners employed, i.e. in urban areas and larger rural Health Centers.

Polish Health Care System does not limit the frequency of consultations and other medical services. Statistically, a person is consulted 6.1 times a year (8.9 times in urban and 2.1 in rural areas); this number includes also specialist's consultations and varies in different provinces from 3.5 to 8.9 (6.9 to 13.1 in urban and 1.3 to 3.1 in rural areas).

3. STRUCTURE OF PRACTICES AND USAGE

In 1,704 urban district ambulatories 9,303 primary care physicians are employed, i.e. on an average 5.5 physicians per ambulatory (2.7 general practitioners, 2.2 pediatricians and 0.55 gynaecologists). In 3,255 rural Health Centers 3,758 physicians are employed, on an average 1.15 in each. Thus urban area ambulatory has always a general practitioner and mostly a pediatrician but not always a full-time gynaecologist. In rural Health Center in most cases there is a full-time general practitioner and a part-time pediatrician and gynaecologist, which means that those physicians can consult patients not every day or/and only a limited number of hours daily.

In urban areas there are also 2,289 district occupational ambulatories employing 3,922 physicians, caring for employees of large industrial enterprises and their families.

The National Health Care System is supported by 408 cooperative and private ambulatories.

4. REMUNERATION

Every employee in Poland is insured together with his unemployed family. The health insurance covers the majority of health care services. Medicines, some medical supplies and orthopaedic equipment are partly (in varying degree) to be paid for.

There is also a possibility of additional individual insurance recompensing days of absence in work due to illness and not recompensing health care service.

Unemployed patients and foreigners from countries not possessing health insurance agreement with Poland pay for all health services. This occurs infrequently in district ambulatories as such patients usually use the services of cooperative or private ambulatories.

Only Emergency Health Care is more often used by such patients. Employed Polish patients may also be treated outside National Health Care System paying for all services.

5. STRUCTURE OF PATIENTS

5.1 The scope of health care services depends in Poland on patient's condition and needs only. It does not depend on a kind of insurance because there is only one type of obligatory national health insurance in Poland.

5.2 Whenever severe illness is diagnosed the patient is hospitalized. The district physician consults the patient at home or in the ambulatory, gives hospitalization order and ambulance transportation order if necessary.

If there is no need for hospitalization the patient is treated at home. For diagnostic purposes there is a possibility of performing some laboratory tests or ECG examination in patient's home. A nurse comes and performs treatment prescribed, the physician visits the patient at home during his visiting hours as often as he considers necessary. On physician's order a social care nurse from the ambulatory and/or the Polish Red Cross sister takes care of the patient. This last service is not a medical but a housekeeping one (shopping, cleaning, cooking, etc.). Similar procedure is observed in chronic cases but the service is rather less intense.

According to statistics presented earlier, most frequent are pulmonary diseases, skeletal and muscular diseases, cardiac and cardiovascular ones, hypertension, gastric and duodenal ulcer, and neuroses.

5.3 Laboratory investigations in primary care are limited and comprise basic biochemistry and hematology. There is also possible an X-ray examination, ECG and in some cases USG.

Pharmacotherapy is limited by medicine availability and costs, as some patients pay 30 % of the medicine price. In principle, every pharmacy should possess all medicines from the official list (about 2,000) and only such medicines can be dispensed. Other medicines may be available at specially designed pharmacies.

Lesser diagnostic and therapeutic procedures can be carried out in primary care units. However, in such cases a patient is directed mostly to a specialist within an ambulatory or in a hospital. There is a full possibility of rehabilitation in special physicotherapeutic units.

There is no rule limiting a patient in his contacts with the health care or a physician in his both diagnostic and therapeutic decisions. According to data given earlier living in rural areas naturally limits patient-physician contacts.

6. ACCOUNTING

Polish physician is a state functionary paid for all performed services. There is no general documentation concerning accounting. If necessary, medical documentation may serve as index of physician's activity.

An urban general practitioner consults mostly 4 patients hourly, unless it is the first consultation which naturally takes more time. A visit at home takes usually 20 to 30 minutes. The number of patients consulted is noted by the registration desk and passed monthly to the Integrated Health Care Center Director's Office, from where it passes for statistical purposes to the Provincial Physician's Office and to the Ministry of Health.

7. MEDICAL DOCUMENTATION

Medical documentation in primary care is obligatory but scarce. It is limited to a short note concerning patient's complaints, abnormalities found in doctor's examination, laboratory investigations and specialist's consultations. A short note is made each time the patient is consulted.

Physician's orders and the duration of a sick-leave are noted. The sick-leave certificate is given on a special document (L 4) stating duration and cause (in code) of inability to work.

All physician's notes, with consultant's decisions (originals) and laboratory investigation findings are stored in special envelopes at the registration desk. A patient's envelope is passed to a physician if he is supposed to consult the patient either in the ambulatory or at home. After the visit the envelope is returned to the registration desk.

A special documentation is used in special programs for some diseases, when the physician calls the patient regularly for a check-up examination and makes a more formal note about the course of a disease. Special events such as patient's fainting or instant hospitalization are documented too.

The envelopes contain also patient's documentation necessary for sanatory treatment and information of patient's hospital treatment.

There are some diseases of which occurence specialistic department have to be informed, e.g. tuberculosis, veneral diseases, cancers.

8. NON-GOVERNMENTAL ORGANIZATIONS AND PROFESSIONAL BODIES

Primary care physicians associate voluntarily within the Polish Medical Society and in specialistic Scientific Medical Societies.

9. STATUS OF COMPUTER SUPPORT IN THE COUNTRY

There are no computers implemented directly to primary care anywhere in Poland.

10. TRENDS AND FUTURE DEVELOPMENTS OF ASSISTANCE OF COMPUTERS IN HEALTH CARE SYSTEMS

The importance of medical informatics is appreciated in Poland but the advance in this field is slow. Since 1982 the Ministry of Health has founded a specialistic informatic unit within the Programming Department.

In 1980 there was founded the Department of Medical Informatics within the Institute of Biocybernetics of Polish Academy of Sciences. This Department cooperates with the Ministry of Health and with Health Care Service units. During the first five years some investigations concerning the application of computers in a wide range of problems connected with health care were carried out in the Department. Some of them concerned the primary care.

The investigations aimed for the greater part at computer support of a general practitioner in his medical activity.

As a result we have some types of experimental computer systems, e.g. the computer system of registration service for a typical outpatient clinic, the computer system of description of patient's condition, the computer system for cooperation between a physician and a laboratory unit, computer-aided diagnostic and therapeutic systems.

Besides economic and technical difficulties slowing down the introduction of computer support of physicians, there are also serious psychological and communication barriers. The physician should be able to communicate directly with the computer, but using alpha-numeric keyboards does not seem to be the ideal solution.

The research concerning computer applications is carried out in the mentioned Department as well as in some regional health care departments with recently increased intensity. Their purpose is introducing computers in some hospitals and ambulatories within the next five years. At the same time computers will be introduced into management of chosen Integrated Health Care Centers and also on provincial level and in the Ministry. This work is concentrated mostly on computer systems for finance (salaries), employment and for documentation of patient's movement within the health care system.

ACHIEVEMENTS AND FURTHER TASKS OF THE HEALTH AND SOCIAL SERVICES IN DEVELOPING THE ADVANCED SOCIALIST SOCIETY IN THE GERMAN DEMOCRATIC REPUBLIC

D. Panzer, * B. Schirmer, ** H. Weihrauch

MR Dr.sc.med. D. Panzer, Institut für Medizinische Statistik und Datenverarbeitung, 1134 Berlin, Nöldnerstraße 34-36

*OMR Dr.sc.med. B. Schirmer, Ministerium für Gesundheitswesen, 1020 Berlin, Rathausstraße 3

**Doz.Dr.sc.oec. H. Weihrauch, Institut für Informatik und Biomathematik, 1080 Berlin, Schumannstraße 20-21

In 1971 the tasks for developing the advanced socialist society of the GDR were laid down.
The main objective of the five-year plan was "the further improvement of the material and cultural standard of living of the people on the basis of a high rate of development in socialist production, grater efficiency, scientific and technological progress and a higher degree of productivity" (1).

This long-term economic objective which is closely related to the requirements of the economic basic law of socialism made it clear that in our socialist society "economy is a means to an end, namely a means to the increasingly better meeting of the growing material and cultural needs of the working people" (1). According to Wetzstein (1980), a new assessment of our health policy was made in the light of our overall policy since the increasingly better meeting of the needs for medical and social care is directly related to the purpose of socialism which is guaranteeing to the people "the unrestrained development and application of their physical and intellectual abilities ...".

The starting point for defining the tasks of the health service was that it is of immediate importance to our citizens' physical and mental well-being and personal happiness (1).
Between 1971 and 1975, the resources available for our medical and social services had been more than doubled and the intensified reconstruction and modernization of our health facilities was begun. This marked the beginning of a long-term orientation towards a more rapid improvement of the material and technological prerequisites of the work performed in the health sector (4).

An important measure for the implementation of our combined economic and social policy has been the Joint Decree by the Politbureau of the Central Committee of the Socialist Unity Party of Germany (SED), the Council of Ministers of the GDR and the National Executive of the Confederation of Free German Trade Unions of 25 September 1973.
The aim of this Decree was the improvement of the health care of the people and also the improvement of the working and living conditions of the personnel in the health and social services.

In the Decree it is stated among others:
"The concern for the physical and mental well-being of the people is an essential element of the programme of social policies adopted by the 8th Party Congress of the SED" (3).

The demand was to provide assistance to our health workers that will help them in performing their important work; to place the health workers and to allocate resources and funds for repair work in such a way that priority is given to developing those sectors of medical practice which provide continuous care to the people and are most frequently utilized by them for the prevention, diagnosis and treatment of diseases (1). The essential feature of the Decree of 1973 was, as stated by Wetzstein (1980), the new and greater importance placed upon the health and social care of the people in its overall societal context. As a result, priority was given to further developing primary ambulatory medical care. Chief importance was first given to the rapid development of the specialties "General Medicine" and "Paediatrics" as well as "Gynaecology" and "Stomatology".

The emphasis was placed on the construction and extension of policlinics and smaller ambulatory facilities as well as on the expansion of ambulatory medical care in working-class districts and industrial centres. Specialized medical care should be, above all, strengthened by expanding the specialties intensive therapy, long-term maintenance haemodialysis, accident surgery, child surgery and urology.

In highly specialized medical care, the emphasis was placed on developing cardiosurgery, neurosurgery and kidney transplantation services. The planned placement of medical graduates in surgical specialties had been also envisaged for the specialties of anaesthesiology and neurology/psychiatry. In addition to reaching these goals the aim was to maintain and further develop the standard achieved in mother and child health care and in dispensary care (i.e. follow-up care). The increased involvement of general practitioners in these processes was a planned development.

Since 1971 the following achievements have been made:

- Older hospitals, policlinics, physicians' offices, créches, and old people's and nursing homes have been reconstructed and improved bringing about better conditions for care and treatment.

- There had been an increase in the amount of preventive services as, for instance, in occupational health care, mother and child health care, child dental care, and there was an increase in the scope of preventive examinations for the early detection of cervical cancer, etc.

- The numbers of persons working in the health service and the medical density have been steadily increasing so that there now is one physician per 450 inhabitants, while in 1949 the medical density was one physician per 1.430 inhabitants. There are altogether more than 540.000 people working in the GDR health and social services.

- The capacities available for medical and social care have been steadily increasing. For the year 1985 increases are planned of more than 400 medical and 220 dental places of work in ambulatory care, of 12.700 places in créches and of more than 4.500 places in old peoples and nursing homes and also of 1.140 places for physically and mentally disabled children. There will be an additional 12.300 health workers, so that by the end of the five-year plan from 1981 to 1985, a total of 20.200 medical and 10.130 dental places of work will be available. This will, as Schirmer (1985) stated, call for the still better implementation of the family physician concept, especially in the big cities and industrial centres, because it is of great importance to the higher effectiveness of our work.

- Medical and social care is being increasingly appreciated as an essential prerequisite for the harmonious physical and mental development of the people, for developing the individual's personality and efficiency, and improving the capacity for work of the working people (Seidel, 1985).

- Special importance is given to further developing primary medical care and especially family physician care. This is in line with our social policy to always solve those problems first which concern the great majority of our population (Seidel, 1985).

It is our aim to provide good medical care to the citizens in the community and in enterprises without causing too much waiting time to them and to exert an influence on the universal development of stable relations and confidence between the family or occupational health physician and the citizen and on the better implementation of the principles of preventive health and the adoption of healthful life practices.

In the health facilities our health workers are engaged in steadily increasing the quality and effectiveness of their work, while also trying to achieve an even more favourable cost-benefit relationship creating, as Harig (1985) stated, health and efficiency, social security, personal well-being and happiness of the people, at the same time preserving and improving their capacity for work.

In our national economy, this process is, in general, reflected by a national system of accounting and statistics which is also of basic importance to the facilities of the health and social services.
The regulation on accounting and statistics as well as the instruction pertaining to the reliable and complete data provision and to data protection in accounting and statistics which will come into force on 1 January 1986 will be providing a body of legal measures which is to extend the uniform system of accounting and statistics having been in existence since 1966 and to take account of the development of our socialist society. We understand by accounting and statistics the uniform system of collecting, processing, storing, reporting and interpreting of numerical information needed for the management, planning, accounting and control of our national economy in accordance with our main objective. The main responsibility for the national management of accounting and statistics has the Central Statistical Office as an executive body of the Council of Ministers. It is responsible for devising the further development and for coordinating all elements of accounting and statistics. The director of the Central Statistical Office is responsible for instructing the state bodies. Centralized reportings are the responsibility of the Central Statistical Office. In addition to the centralized reportings special reportings with regard to specific questions of the health sector are carried out. Among the special reportings are those needed for health management and planning purposes which are proposed by the health and social services and approved by the Central Statistical Office. The Ministry of Health and the Institute of Medical Statistics and Data Processing have the main responsibility for rationalization, documentation and organization of data provision for the special reportings which can be subdivided into:

- medical and social care,

- hygiene and occupational hygiene,

- facilities and services, utilization of personnel and material resources,

- education and continuing education of the health personnel,

- drug provision, health technology, material and technological basis.

The responsibility of the central administrative level is to guarantee the uniformly run and organized process of all health facilities of our country. For this purpose the Institute of Medical Statistics and Data Processing of the Ministry of Health was founded as a guiding centre earlier this year. An information about this new institute was already given at the 6th Congress of EFMI in Helsinki in August 1985 (9).

In the counties (Bezirke) there are Medical Statistical Offices which have to guarantee the information handling, organization and statistical analysis in the county. The founding of Medical Statistical Offices in the districts (Kreise) is being continued, and in the health facility the responsibility for statistics rests with the book-keeper or the sector for economy and planning. The regulations passed by the Ministry are laid down in information orders, catalogues of approved reportings and approved indices. In these documents the responsibilities in the field of statistics are clearly defined for each level of management. The most important task of the information system is to secure the rapid availability of indices necessary for operational management in the districts and facilities and for the medium-term and long-term planning at the district and ministry levels. Information for the assessment of the health status of the population is becoming increasingly important. Based upon the potential of electronic data processing, at the end of the 1970ies it was begun to systematize information related to health facilities, i.e. information on capacities, profile, expenditure and services of the facilities, while also incorporating data on patients and health personnel, and to process them by computer avoiding to a great degree hitherto existing shortcomings as double collection, insufficient timeliness, high amount of work. The result was the designing and gradual putting into practice of the report of the facility which is to gradually replace the hitherto isolated data reportings pertaining to health facilities by a number of compatible segments of the report of the facility. This replacement is, as stated by Panzer, Wolf and Ziesemer (1983), taking place in the following sectors where there are computer-assisted partial projects:

- insurance carriers and finances,

- health personnel,

- crèches and permanent homes,

- in-patient facilities,

- ambulatory dental facilities,

- ambulatory facilities,

- old people's and nursing homes.

In a second stage such elements as the material and technical sector as well as dispensary care facilities, etc. will be included. The combination with morbidity statistics which are primarily provided by registers and our in-patient record project is envisaged for the future. These stages will be realized in accordance with the further development of the availability of computer technology in the counties, districts and, above all, in the health facilities as far as to the place where the medical activity is performed.

A register of the facility has been designed as a means of integration for the report of the facility which reflects the entire institutional structure of the health and social services. While in all facility-related reportings the 8-digit number of the facility has to appear on the basic records, in all person-related reportings the personal identification number or an abridged form of it is used. Due to its structure and the organizational projects, the report of the facility secures not only the operational flow of information within the facility but also the flow of information within the information pyramid as far as to the Institute of Medical Statistics and Data Processing. The prerequisites for achieving an up-to-date information provision are that the data are acquired decentrally, i.e. in the facility as far as to the county level, that the checking and correction of the data are made in the county and that first evaluations and feedback to the facility are made.

The central handling of the project is then made in our Institute by processing the data of the counties. This project design is made possible by the technological development and is being fully supported by the facilities, the districts and counties since they can all profit by the more rapid provision of information. This process is being promoted by the installation of electronic computer equipment in the statistical offices of the counties, in the large hospitals, in selected policlinics as well as by the gradual equipment of medical work stations with personal computers. This development is also set out in the principles for the utilization of electronic data processing in the sector coming under the responsibility of the Ministry of Health for the period 1986 - 1990 which have been adopted in September 1985.

The targets for the further utilization of electronic data processing in the health service are:

- the provision of information for management and planning purposes according to the needs of the users to be used in decision making;
- the utilization of modern computer solutions in the information system for management and planning;
- the increase in user friendliness and acceptance of the computer projects;
- the development of modern methods and technologies for the further decentralization of data processing.

In the coming years, medical statistics will have the following main tasks:

- to reflect changes in the health status of the population,
- to reflect the quality and efficiency of medical care,
- to assist management in formulating and implementing the plan and in measuring its execution,
- to provide up-to-date information on facilities, services and personnel.

Further tasks will be patient-related data processing, data processing in laboratories, medical supply processes, hygiene and occupational health care, support to research and scientific work in the health facilities.

It should also be mentioned that in our research project "Computer-assisted information systems in health facilities" work is performed directly in the health facilities and new solutions to be standardized are being created and that there already is in the counties and health facilities a considerable potential of qualified personnel actively supporting and advancing the envisaged process. In this way we will succeed in achieving the objectives of our social policy to steadily improve medical and social care.

References

1. Bericht des Zentralkomitees an den VIII. Parteitag der Sozialistischen Einheitspartei Deutschlands, (1971) Dietz Verlag, Berlin

2. Direktive des VIII. Parteitages der SED zum Fünfjahrplan für die Entwicklung der Volkswirtschaft der DDR 1971-1975 (1971) Dietz Verlag, Berlin

3. Weitere Maßnahmen zur Durchführung des sozialpolitischen Programms des VIII. Parteitages der SED. Gemeinsamer Beschluß des Politbüros des ZK der SED, dem Ministerrates der DDR und des Bundesvorstandes des FDGB vom 25. September 1973 in: Neues Deutschland vom 27. Sept. 1973,

4. Büttner L, Meyer B , Wetzstein E (1980) Gesundheitspolitik - Aufgaben und Traditionen. VEB Gustav Fischer Verlag, Jena, p. 131

5. Harig E (1985) Stets und überall ein hohes Niveau der medizinischen Betreuung, Humanitas 25:3 Heft 15

6. Panzer D, Wolf K, Ziesemer H (1983) Prinzipien des Aufbaus eines einheitlichen Berichtswesens am Beispiel des Einrichtungsberichtes Vortrag

7. Schirmer B (1985) Auf dem Weg zum XI. Parteitag - unser Plan 1985 Humanitas 25:1 Heft 1

8. Seidel K (1985) Vorbereitung des XI. Parteitages der SED- unser aller Sache Humanitas 25:1 Heft 14

9. Schirmer B, Panzer D (1985) The Systems of Medical Statistics in the GDR and Targets upto 1990 in F.H. Roger, Grönroos, P, Tervo-Pellika R and O'Moore R (eds.): Lecture Notes in Medical Informatics 25, Springer Verlag, Berlin-Heidelberg-New York-Tokyo 309-313

Primary Health Care in Hungary

P. Simon[1] and A. Naszlady[2]

[1]Organization, Planning and Information Center, Ministry of Health, Arany J.u.6-8, Budapest H-1361
and
[2]National Institute of Pulmonology
Pihenő u. 1, Budapest H-1529, Hungary

INTRODUCTION

Social insurance is extended to everybody who is an Hungarian citizen and lives in Hungary. To be insured is by right of Hungarian citizenship. Social insurance matters are handled by Social Insurance Center of the Trade Unions.

During illness the patient is entitled to sick leave. The amount paid as sick pay is 65-75 per cent of his(her) wages. In case of hospitalization the patient receives half the sick pay otherwise due (but the family breadwinner receives 80 per cent).

A working woman receives sick pay also when she has to stay at home to nurse her child under 3 years of age. A working woman is entitled to 10 weeks paid maternity leave. New mothers are also paid a maternity grant for each child and receive baby outfits as well. Additional supports are: widow's pension, orphans' allowance, disablement allowance, funeral aid.

1. STRUCTURE OF PRIMARY HEALTH CARE

1.1 Principles

Two main or guiding principles determine the system of health care. First: territorial integration of health care units; second: progressive medical care management.

Territorial integration means the operation of health institutions and curative facilities are supplied, controlled, and coordinated by the health administrative department of the local council. The tasks of local public health and of health care are performed by health centers (united inpatient-outpatient institutions) which consist of hospital(s), outpatient department(s), dispensaries, and offices for doctors of the primary health care system (district doctors).

The principle of progressive medical care management means that the units of health services are arranged in a hierarchical

---

[1]Director of the center

[2]Professor of Medicine, Head of Cardiopulmonary Dept.

order of specialty so that the more complicated the diagnostic and/or therapeutical problem, the higher the level of specialized institution is available for the patient.(Fig.1.)

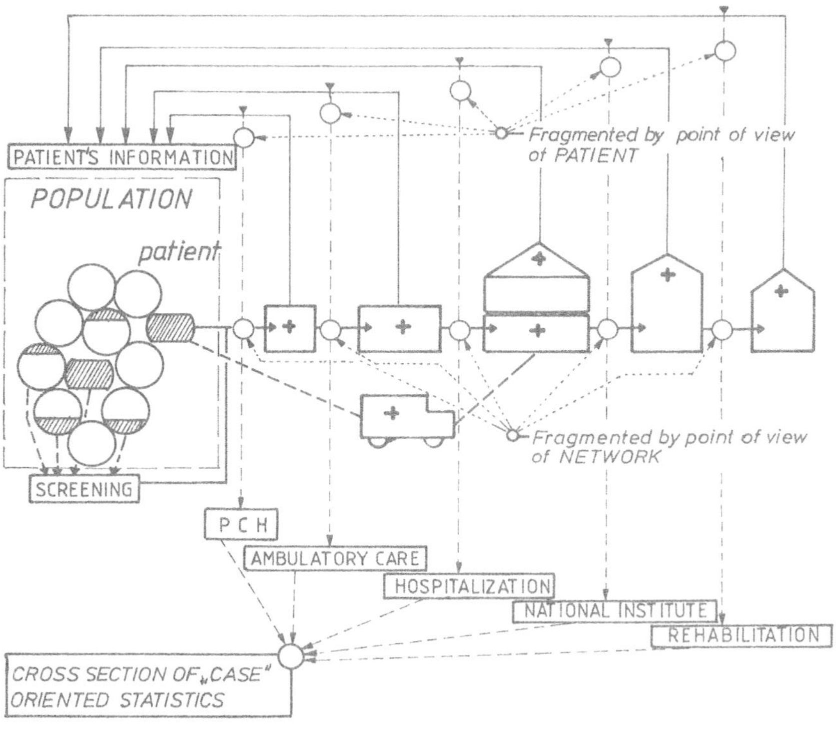

Fig.1. Scheme of case-oriented information process

The rank order of this system extends from primary medical care through specialized ambulatory care - outpatient department - hospital (municipal) - country hospital - university clinic - specialized regional center - as far as national institutes of different specialties.

1.2. Organization and personnel of primary health care

Population can electively get contact first with any of the following health services: district doctor, district paediatrician, doctor of school health care, district dentist, doctor of enterprise-based health service, doctors of dispensaries for different special cares (for pregnants, for venereal diseases, for tbc patients etc). All of these services are not accessible in country side where the district doctor's duty is to provide most of them. So district doctors are really general practitioners (GP). In addition GP has to take care of quality control of foodstuffs, water, health information and education of people in catchment area. GP's duty is combating against infectious diseases (quarantine, vaccinations, immunizations etc.) and enforce primary prevention in every respect as far as possible.

The network of district doctors is controlled by both the health administrative department of the local council and by the territorial Health Center. In this organization the whole population is being provided with sufficient health care, sometimes and/or somewhere even with some overlapping too. (Fig.2.)

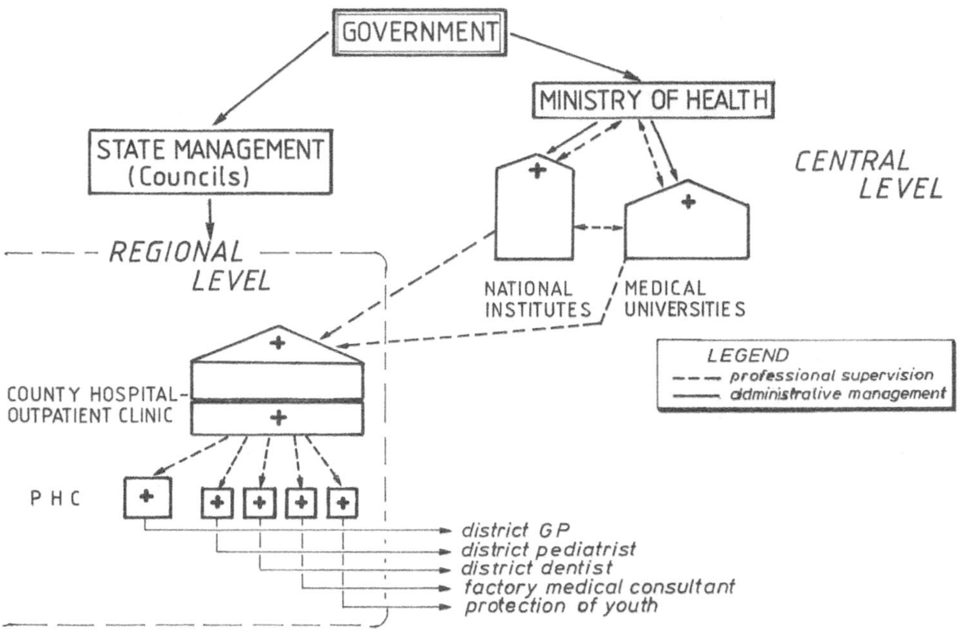

Fig.2. The structure of curative and preventive care in Hungary

The number of medical doctors was 34000 and the number of district doctors was 4248 in 1984 (Simon and Kövesi 1985). The doctor - to - adult persons ratio in catchment areas is on the average 2000 people / GP. (Table 1.)

Table 1. Data of curative-preventive care

	1970	1984
Number of GP districts	3 796	4 374
Number of district GP	3 646	4 248
Number of paediatric districts	606	1 260
Number of district pediatrist	589	1 205
Average number of inhabitants per district (GP+pediatrist)	2 444	1 955
Number of protection of youth	218	165
Daily consulting hours at factory doctors	5 449	11 039
Number of factory medical consultants	1 363	2 163

GP is helped by an administrative worker and by one nurse.

1.3. Expenditure

For primary health care separately costs are not calculated. The total social and health care expenditure is 4,8 per cent of the national revenue. (Hungarian Stat. 1983.)

2. STRUCTURE OF POPULATION

In Hungary about 10 million people are living. The population density per square km is 107, one of the more densily populated countries in Europe. Approximately 20 per cent of inhabitants live in the capital, 22 per cent in the other towns and 58 per cent in villages. In Table 2. the population subdivided by age and sex is presented from 1941 till 1985. In Table 3.the death rates per 100 000 population for leading causes of death is given comparing data of the last fifty years.

Table 2. Distribution of population (%)

	Years	0-14	15-39	40-59	60-69	70-X
man	1941	26,8	41,3	21,6	6,3	4,0
	1949	26,2	38,9	24,1	6,7	4,1
	1960	26,9	37,2	23,6	7,6	4,7
	1970	22,4	38,2	24,3	9,5	5,6
	1980	23,2	37,4	24,7	7,9	6,8
	1985	22,9	37,5	24,5	8,0	7,1
woman	1941	25,6	40,0	23,7	6,8	4,3
	1949	23,6	38,6	25,2	7,9	4,7
	1960	24,0	36,3	24,5	9,1	6,1
	1970	19,9	35,9	25,4	10,8	8,0
	1980	20,6	34,2	25,8	9,4	10,0
	1985	20,3	33,8	25,2	9,7	11,0

	Years	0-14	15-39	40-59	60-69	70-X
total	1941	26,0	40,1	22,7	6,5	4,7
	1949	24,9	38,8	24,7	4,2	4,4
	1960	25,4	36,8	24,0	8,4	5,4
	1970	21,1	37,0	24,8	10,2	6,9
	1980	21,7	36,1	25,3	8,7	8,2
	1985	21,6	35,6	24,8	8,9	9,1

Table 3. Mortality rates per 100 000 population

CAUSES OF DEATH	1970	1983
Heart and hypertensive diseases	357,8	380,4
Malignant neoplasms	215,3	265,9
Cerebrovascular diseases	169,0	221,4
Arteriosclerosis	72,8	108,1
Accidents (total)	54,4	72,2
Bronchitis, enphysema and asthma	21,8	51,3
Suicide and self-inflected injury	34,8	45,9
Chronic liver disease and cirrhosis	12,9	39,2
Diabetes mellitus	8,1	19,3
Certain types of chronic diseases of the kidney	7,4	5,4
Certain conditions originating in the perinatal period	32,0	12,7
Influenza and pneumonia	27,7	19,6
Tuberculosis (including late consequences as well)	19,3	10,2
Other infectious and parasitic diseases	7,6	2,7

3. STRUCTURE OF PRACTICES AND USAGE

The GP plays a central role in the health care system in Hungary. If the GP considers further diagnostic examination and/or therapeutical intervention or any other specialised medical aid to be necessary, he sends the patient to the nearest upper level of progressive care with a letter of referral. After having finished their interventions the specialists send the results and their suggestions in written form back to that GP who sent the patient to them previously. In towns it is possible and becomes more and more common that GP's offices are settled in the same building where specialised ambulatory care is also functioning. This makes it easier to access consultations both for patients and for doctors. However, it does not mean that those GPs would be in cooperation to each other forming a team or group practices. Some data on patients' turnover is shown in Table 4.

Table 4. Data of patient turnover at the service of district GPs

NUMBER OF PATIENT CONSULTATIONS	PATIENTS VISITED IN THEIR HOMES	PATIENTS SENT TO SPECIALIST CONSULTATIONS	PATIENTS SENT TO HOSPITAL	PATIENTS UNDER A LONG TERM CARE
PATIENT TURNOVER OF DISTRICT G Ps				
38 433 704	4 426 716	2 399 962	211 209	1 206 942
ANNUAL TURNOVER PER DISTRICT				
8787	1012	549	48	253
ANNUAL TURNOVER OF PATIENTS PER 100 INHABITANTS				
360,6	41,5	22,5	2,0	11,3

4. REMUNERATION

Contributions to meet the costs of social insurance are borne by the employers in full and the Government covers the remainder expenses from the taxation. Employees have to pay only a so-called "old age contribution" which progressively increases with the amount of total wages. Hungarian physicians - all of them, not only GP - are state functionaries paid with fix salaries irrespective to the amount of services they performed. There is no capitation fee for the doctors.

5. STRUCTURE OF PATIENTS

5.1. Insurance status

As has been mentioned above, Hungarian people have obligatory health insurance by right of citizenship.

5.2. Morbidity spectrum

The knowledge about the morbidity of general population is very limited. There are data collected about the causes and number of days of sick leave (Fig.3.). Respiratory diseases, cardiovascular diseases, accidents and musculo-skeletal diseases are the leading categories.

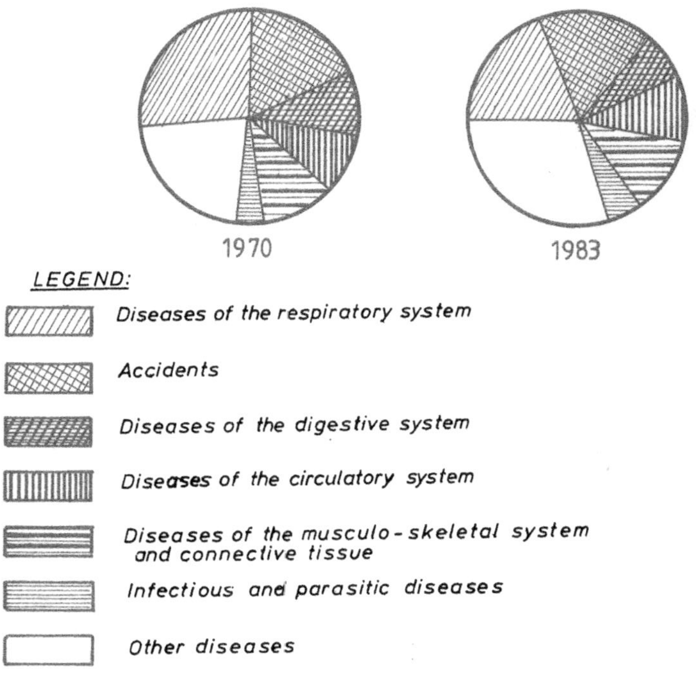

Fig.3. The causes and number of days of sick leave

5.3. Treatment spectrum

There is no limitation for physicians to prescribe medicines being on official lists. It is also possible to have special drugs imported if needed.

6. ACCOUNTING

General practitioners are not obliged to register costs, expenses or any financial documents.

7. MEDICAL DOCUMENTATION

Medical documentation is obligatory in primary medical care. Usually it consists of A/5 size cards with short notices about patient's complaints, alternations in physical findings and interventions carried out and/or advised. In addition a diary is written for summarizing the numbers of daily visits either at office or at patient's home. The mostly controlled documentation is the sick leave diary.

8. ORGANIZATIONS AND PROFESSIONAL BODIES

Primary health care physicians may associate within their own society and/or in any of Hungarian medical societies.

9. STATUS OF COMPUTER SUPPORT IN THE COUNTRY

9.1. Types

At the level of primary health care there is no official support for installation of computers. There are, however, five medical regional centers officially pointed out to develop medical informatics and computerization for different sectors of the health care system.

Each center has its own special task: a regional, a hospital, an educational, a research and a centralized statistical computerized system have to be worked out. These centers are already operating for at least ten years and a lot of programs are constructed and delivered by them.

9.2. Penetration

The transportability of this software, however, is very difficult because a new tendency is observable in computerizations: a great rise in numbers of personal computers and their penetration into the health care system is inevitable. The adaptations of software have been initiated, but technical development seems to be more rapid than software production could keep abreast to it.

9.3. Problems

Informatically speaking our system is "care-oriented", which results in a lot of disadvantages. Some of them are:
- it is impossible to follow the patient,
- it is impossible to study the evolution of diseases,
- GP became - in too many instances - a dispatcher who only directed but not cured the patients,
- a lot of superfluous parallelism took place by sending the patient to various consultations without continuous documentation,
- it is impossible to obtain reliable morbidity data.

10. TRENDS

In order to solve or avoid these problems, a new "patient-oriented" information system is now developing based on the nation wide established personal identity number. To achieve this aim and establishing the new, more effective information system a health state determination of the general population was needed at first. (Fig.4.)

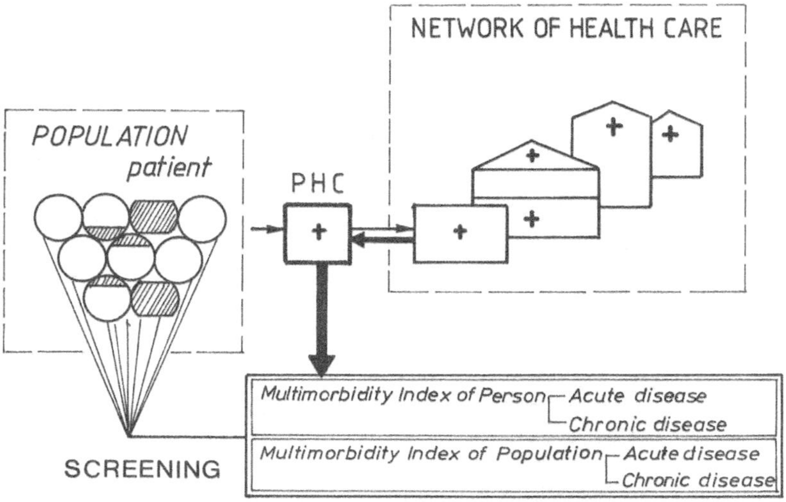

Fig.4. Indicators for observation in the patient-oriented information systems

Purpose: 1 To assert the health status of population to identify groups in the need of
- care
- treatment
- active surveillance

2 To analyse efficiency of the network (optimum:few sick people-many healthy of contorol)

3 To get a more precise knowledge about needs and requirements to be met by health service (primary needs, individual and social requirement)

Conditions: 1 Strengthening of PHC-function

2 Interactive user-friendly (microcomputer) systems

This is being done by a population mass-screening, the results of which are passed to GP. The multiphasic mass-screening is organized together with obligatory anti-tbc chest X-ray screening (Directives 1985). It has been rarified from yearly to 2-years repetition, having taken into account the decrease in tbc cases, the analysis of efficacy (Seelentag 1979).

"Multiphasic" means that the screening is extended to five disease categories as follows (with prevalence in per cent in parenthesis): cardiovascular incl. hypertension (19%), chronic respiratory diseases (6%), diabetes mellitus (2%), chronic renal diseases (3%), tumor (especially breast cc. or gynecol. cc. - 2%) (Naszlady 1985).

More than 2 million people have been passed through this screening until now.

Regarding documentation at population level we are studying the usability of a patient's memory card system (SANINFORM Pat. Reg.[x])[3]. The system consists of 3 main parts: a data entry and retrieval unit, a ROM adapter to house TV set, a data storage ROM (suitable for personal wear).

Screening and individual data storage ROM integrated in a patient-oriented information system are the aims we are working for in the nearest future.

[x3] invented by Naszlady, Simon, Gulyás, Winkler, Szöllős in LICENCIA Co BUDAPEST Pf207 H-1368

References

Directives to further development of social welfare in the 7th five-year-plan period (1985)
Eds Hungarian Ministry of Health Budapest p 46

Hungarian Statistical Booklet (1983) Statisztikai Kiadó Vállalat Budapest p 98

Naszlady A (1985) Studies on cardiopulmonary system as a unit (scientific research report in Hungarian) in: Results of Researches granted by Hungarian Ministry of Health Budapest vol I. pp 159-160

Simon P, Kövesi E (1985) Development of Hungarian Health Service in Hungarian. Eds ESZTIK BUDAPEST p 11

Seelentag W (1979) Evaluating the role of X-ray diagnosis in public health WHO Chronicle 33:53-55

AUTHOR INDEX

SUBJECT INDEX

ADDRESSES OF THE AUTHORS

Assimacopoulos, André	M.D. Division d'Informatique Hôpital Cantonal Universitaire CH-1211 Genéve 4 / Switzerland
Dostal, Clibor	M.D., Ph.D. Clinical Department Research Institute of Rheumatology Naslupi 4 CSSR-12026 Praha 2 / Czechoslovakia
Dumont, Francois	M.D. Unaformec-France 311, rue Lecourbe F-75015 Paris / France
Gallois, Pierre	M.D. Unaformec-France 311, rue Lecourbe F-75015 Paris / France
Geus, C.A. de	Dept. of Medical Informatics and Statistics Rijksuniversiteit Limburg POB 616 NL-6200 MD Maastricht / The Netherlands
Hasman, Arie	Prof. Dept. of Medical Informatics and Statistics Rijksuniversiteit Limburg POB 616 NL-6200 MD Maastricht / The Netherlands
Janecki, Jerzy	Doc. Dr. med. Samodzielna Pracownia Informatyki Kliniczney IBIB PAN ul. Rutkowskiego 12 PL-00-020 Warszawa / Poland
Jokinen, Yrjö	M.D. Computing Centre University of Kuopio POB 6 SF-70211 Kuopio / Finland
Leimanis, A.	Hälso- och sjukvårdsförvaltningen POB 9099 S-102 72 Stockholm / Sweden
McLachlan, Richard	Prof. Department of Family Medicine Family Medicine Centre of Queen's University 220 Bagot Street POB 8888 Kingston / Canada K7L5E9

Möhr, Jochen R.	Prof. Institut für Medizin. Dokumentation, Statistik und Datenverarbeitung der Universität Im Neuenheimer Feld 325 D-6900 Heidelberg 1 / F.R. Germany
Naszlady, Attila	Prof. National Institute of Pulmonology Cardiopulmonary Department Pihenö u. 1 H-1529 Budapest / Hungary
O'Moore, Rory R.	M.D. St. James's Hospital Dept. of Biochemistry Central Pathology Laboratory POB 580 IRL-Dublin 8 / Ireland
Panzer, Doris	MR Dr. sc. med. Institut für Medizininische Statistik und Datenverarbeitung Nöldnerstraße 34 - 36 DDR-3134 Berlin / German Dem. Rep.
Peterson, Hans	M.D. Hälso- och sjukvårdsförvaltningen POB 9099 S-102 72 Stockholm / Sweden
Peumans, Willy	Dr. I.C. Systems G. Verwilghensingel 4 B-3500 Hasselt / Belgium
Rosis, Fiorella de	Prof. Health Information Systems Istituto di Scienze dell'Informazione Università Via Mendola 173 I-70100 Bari / Italy
Schirmer, B.	OMR Dr. sc. med. Ministerium für Gesundheitswesen Rathausstraße 3 DDR-1020 Berlin / German Dem. Rep.
Simon, Pál	M.D. Organization, Planning and Information Center Ministry of Health Arany J. u. 6 - 8 H-1361 Budapest / Hungary
Stoddart, Norman	M.B., B.S. St. Wilfried Square UK-Calverton Nottingham NGI 4 6FP / United Kingdom

Struthers, Don

M.D.
Practice Management Plans (Pty) Ltd.
POB 5780
ZA-Johannesburg 2000 / Rep. South Africa

Vuori, Hannu

M.D., Ph.D., M.A.
Chief, Research Promotion
and Development
World Health Organization
Regional Office for Europe
Scherfigsvej 8
DK-2100 Copenhagen / Denmark

Weihrauch, Helmut

Doz. Dr. sc. oec.
Institut für Informatik und
Biomathematik
Humboldt-Universität
Schumannstraße 20 - 21
DDR-1080 Berlin / German Dem. Rep.

Yanagita, Yoichiro

M.D.
Tokyo Maternity Clinic
1-20-8, Sendagaya, Shibuya-ku
J-Tokyo 151 / Japan

Zámková, V.

Dept. of Social Medicine
Medical Faculty
Charles University
CSSR-Prague / Czechoslovakia

Zvárová, J.

Dept. of Social Medicine
Mecial Faculty
Charles University
CSSR-Prague / Czechoslovakia

Lecture Notes in Medical Informatics

Vol. 23: Selected Topics in Image Science. Edited by O. Nalcioglu and Z.-H. Cho. IX, 308 pages. 1984.

Vol. 24: Medical Informatics Europe 1984. Proceedings, 1984. Edited by F.H. Roger, J.L. Willems, R. O'Moore and B. Barber. XXVII, 778 pages. 1984.

Vol. 25: Medical Informatics Europe 1985. Edited by F.H. Roger, P. Grönroos, R. Tervo-Pellikka and R. O'Moore. XVII, 823 pages. 1985.

Vol. 26: Methodical Problems in Early Detection Programmes. Proceedings, 1983. Edited by E. Walter and A. Neiß. VIII, 198 pages. 1985.

Vol. 27: E. Mergenthaler, Textbank Systems. VI, 177 pages. 1985.

Vol. 28: Objective Medical Decision Making. Proceedings, 1985. Edited by D. D. Tsiftsis. VII, 229 pages. 1986.

Vol. 29: System Analysis of Ambulatory Care in Selected Countries. Edited by P. L. Reichertz, R. Engelbrecht and U. Piccolo. VI, 197 pages. 1986.

GPSR Compliance

The European Union's (EU) General Product Safety Regulation (GPSR) is a set of rules that requires consumer products to be safe and our obligations to ensure this.

If you have any concerns about our products, you can contact us on ProductSafety@springernature.com

In case Publisher is established outside the EU, the EU authorized representative is:

Springer Nature Customer Service Center GmbH
Europaplatz 3
69115 Heidelberg, Germany

Batch number: 10704763

Printed by Printforce, the Netherlands